Penthouse Variations on

quickies

Penthouse Variations on

quickies

BY THE EDITORS OF
PENTHOUSE VARIATIONS

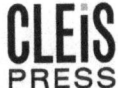

Published in the United States by Cleis Press, an imprint of Start Midnight LLC, 101 Hudson Street, 37th Floor, Suite 3705, Jersey City, New Jersey 07302.

Cover design: Scott Idleman/Blink
Cover Photo: Courtesy of Penthouse Variations Magazine
Text design: Frank Wiedemann
First Edition.
10 9 8 7 6 5 4 3 2 1

Trade paper ISBN: 978-1-62778-194-7
E-book ISBN: 978-1-62778-195-4

Certain materials herein were previously published in *Penthouse Variations* magazine.

CONTENTS

vii   Introduction   *Barbara Pizio*

1   Hot Little Number   *Dante Davidson*

6   The Power of Three   *Emilie Paris*

11   Spank You Later   *Alison Tyler*

16   Hot Stuff   *Priscilla Lawrence*

21   Behind the Curtain   *Bella Dean*

26   Deep Desires   *Christopher Monroe*

31   Corporate Affairs   *Sadie Reynolds*

37   Butterfingers   *Victoria Neilson*

42   Cooking Up Kink   *Sommer Marsden*

48   My Wife's Playmate   *Benjamin Eliot*

53   Meeting the Neighbors   *Lily Aikens*

58   Special Delivery   *Davis Carter*

64   His Bad Girl   *Quinn Gabriel*

69   Come Here Often?   *Marsha Lewis*

74   A Playful Getaway   *Vivian Arias*

80   Boss Lady   *Kitty Winston*

85   A Real Handy Man   *Max Smith*

91   Girl Crush   *Maria Stewart*

96   Hungry for Pleasure   *Laurie Hall*

101   Carnal Cravings   *Marlie Palmer*

106   Welcome to the Neighborhood   *Catherine Murphy*

112   His Wanton Wife   *Sabrina Porter*

117   The Cure for the Common Threeway   *Tucker Wallace*

120   Backdoor Bliss   *Eric Williams*

125   The Office Adonis *Tony Addario*

130   Jessica's Oral Fixation *Patrick Fergusen*

134   Sultry Sex Show *Tawny Webster*

139   His Straying Spouse *Kevin Potter*

144   Spanking Good Fun *Jackie Martise*

149   Taking the Temp *Benjamin Houston*

155   Meeting Her Match *Jewel Rodriguez*

160   The Bling's the Thing *Stella Piazza*

165   Pretty Panties *Melanie Klein*

170   Randy Reunion *Bethany Duggan*

175   Big Spender *Rita Winchester*

180   Hot Head *James Saturne*

185   Dirty Delights *Alice Mueller*

190   Dripping Wet *Hannah Perkins*

195   That Kind of Girl *Jennifer Peters*

200   Corrective Measures *Sam Morris*

205   Sultry Sex Ed *Jenna Lui*

210   Horny Homecoming *Peter McLoughlin*

216   Back to Basics *Penelope Chevalier*

222   Making New Memories *Mitch Rodgers*

228   A Perfect Match *Mark Donohue*

233   Pretty Little Hand-Me-Downs *Angelo Vitale*

239   Doing Things Differently *Sarah Jackson*

244   Taken for a Ride *Vance Peterman*

Introduction

Hot, fast and dirty—those are the sexy hallmarks of the short but sizzling stories from *Penthouse Variations* magazine that compose this collection. *Variations* readers know that there's an undeniable appeal to urgent erotic encounters, in all of their varied forms.

Impromptu adventures embody many people's fantasies of living out their wildest dreams, and Dante Davidson perfectly captures the divine providence of hooking up with an unexpected admirer in "Hot Little Number":

> Her apartment was decorated in a simple, classic style. But she didn't give me much of a tour. The connection between us was simply too strong. When she invited

me out onto her fire escape, I didn't waste a second before kissing her. The chill of the predawn air flowed over us, but the heat we shared robbed me of any need to shiver. She was lovely and light in my arms, her crystalline hair combed clean off her face, her lips painted a rich, dark red. She was all femme without the fatale.

When she put her hand out to stroke my cock, I leaned back against the building and let her. For such a pretty young thing, she definitely knew how to work a man.

In "Hot Stuff," Priscilla Lawrence tells the tale of curious college coeds who go from strangers to lesbian lovers after an off-campus encounter:

In her sunlit apartment, we set down the coffees and our bags and then, before any awkwardness could set in, she was undressing. I leaned against the wall and watched her. She slipped off her yellow V-neck, her sandals, and then she started to work on those painted-on jeans. I couldn't stand the suspense. I came over and helped her, pulling them down myself and going on my knees at the same time. I pressed her up against the arm of her sofa and set my mouth against the front of her panties. These were a lighter yellow than her T-shirt and nearly sheer. I licked her through the fabric and she sighed, letting me know I was on the right track to her pleasure stop.

However, passion isn't limited to first-time lovers, with married couples also having a kinky good time, as in Rita Winchester's "Big Spender":

> Dominic came into the room, flicked my dress up with a practiced hand and began spanking me without a word, alternating strokes—right, left, right, left until my bottom thrummed with heat and blazed with pain. I found that I'd scooched myself forward and was grinding myself against the very edge of the table, trying desperately to get off.
>
> Dom's hand stilled and moved away. "Knock it off."
>
> Again, I froze. I was panting; I could hear my own ragged breath.
>
> His finger drove into me from behind, and my pussy made a slick, wet sound when he entered me. I gasped, moving back to encourage him to drive his finger deeper. He added a second, flexed them once, withdrew, and then spread my own juices over my tingling clit before quickly pulling his hand away.

These skillful writers demonstrate that scrimping on time does not mean sacrificing pleasure. Their steamy tales of sudden sex get straight to the point, delivering bite-sized, blissful escapades to inspire your own sensual fun.

Barbara Pizio
Executive Editor, *Penthouse Variations*

Hot Little Number

DANTE DAVIDSON

"What's a dame got to do to get a drink around here?"

I don't pick up girls every night of the week. I could. I know that. As a bartender at one of the hipper clubs in our city, I definitely get hit on several times an evening. But usually, I wind up alone at home, watching old black-and-white movies on TV and drinking a beer by myself. I don't consider myself jaded—but at forty-five, I've seen my share of human behavior. Drama is not my thing. I long for the high-end interactions I devour in the movies from the '40s, the quick-talking banter between witty characters.

"A dame?" I echoed.

"That's what I said," the customer repeated as she settled herself on the corner bar stool. She was captivating. Her birch-blonde hair was off her face in a neat ponytail. She had on a sleek black turtleneck and small diamond studs. In the club filled with plunging necklines and serious glitter, she stood out like a white rose in a sea of dandelions.

"Whiskey. On the rocks."

I knew exactly how old she was because I carded her before her first drink. I had twenty years on her, and I wondered if she knew that as she spent every moment I was free flirting with me.

Throughout the evening, I grew more and more enamored of her. She had a witty sense of humor Bette Davis would have been jealous of, and a half smile that made me want to lean right over the bar and bite her bottom lip. When I made some mention of my favorite black-and-white film, with stars who were young seventy-five years ago, she practically knocked me off my feet by quoting one of the lines.

"How do you know movies like that?" I asked.

"Not everyone fell for *Twilight*," she said, and I liked her even more.

I was sad when she brought out her wallet to pay, and I told her the drink was on the house. She smiled and waved, and when I went to pick up her glass and napkin, I saw that she'd written her name— *Giselle*—and phone number along with the words: *I stay up late.*

I called as soon as I got off, and she gave me directions to her house.

"I'm twenty years older than you," I told her on the phone, so we would be on the same page.

"Older men know how to treat ladies right," she said, and I made it my mission to do exactly that.

When she opened the front door, I got the second surprise of the night. Over her black leather sofa was a framed poster from a classic Bogart and Bacall film. So she hadn't been faking. She really *was* into old movies. As I walked into her place, I saw that there were similar posters everywhere.

Her apartment was decorated in a simple, classic style. But she didn't give me much of a tour. The connection between us was simply too strong. When she invited me out onto her fire escape, I didn't waste a second before kissing her. The chill of the predawn air flowed over us, but the heat we shared robbed me of any need to shiver. She was lovely and light in my arms, her crystalline hair combed clean off her face, her lips painted a rich, dark red. She was all femme without the fatale.

When she put her hand out to stroke my cock, I leaned back against the building and let her. For such a pretty young thing, she definitely knew how to work a man. She undid the buckle of my belt and reached into my pants to jack me in her fist. The stars were up above us. There was neon ablaze in the shop windows down the block. I knew most people would be asleep at this hour, but to be sure we didn't disturb anyone, I ushered her back inside.

In less than a minute, we were naked on the plush cream-colored rug in her living room. I marveled at the beauty of her body. She was pale and delicate looking, but deceptively strong. She took charge at first, having me sit down and then sliding into my lap. I felt her wet pussy against my cock, and I wanted to enter her, but we held still for a moment, not moving. I stared at the movie poster over her sofa. I felt as if we were in our own film. We stayed like that, connected without being joined, for as long as I could possibly handle it.

Then I looked into her eyes and said, "That's all I can take. I have to be inside you."

She laughed and pushed up on her thighs, then slotted the head of my cock against her slit and slid back down. The pleasure was instantaneous. I felt light-headed for a moment, then warm all over. She worked me to her own rhythm, and she braced herself with her palms flat on the rug, let her head fall back and sighed. I observed the raw quality of her beauty, the way her small breasts seemed to be begging for me to touch them, the way the hollow of her throat was infinitely graceful. She was so finely boned, so lovely, that I found myself handling her in a softer way than I might normally have stroked a woman.

Giselle was having none of that. She sat upright and looked directly at me, as if having read my thoughts. "I'm no delicate flower," she said, and as if to prove that, she pulled off me and got on her hands and knees on her carpet. She gazed at me over her shoulder and said gruffly, "Fuck me like this. Fuck me doggie-style."

Okay, so the heroines in the late-night movies I love never talk like that. But if they had, they would have sounded exactly like Giselle, I swear. I took her at her word—she no longer seemed so fragile to me—and I got behind her and set my cock against her pussy.

"Now!" she demanded, and that's all I needed to hear. I gripped her hips and thrust forward. Giselle lowered her head and arched, and her very scent seemed to change. The room was filled with the aroma of us fucking. I had never been with a girl who was so quickly aroused, so deeply wet.

Giselle slid one hand between her legs and gave my balls a tug. I groaned and fucked her harder. I could tell when she started to finger her pussy, and I removed her hand and replaced her digits with my own. I rubbed her button as I fucked her, and she started urging me on. "Oh fuck—that feels so good. You're making me feel so fucking good."

I loved the way she sounded, the crisp tone of her voice as she let the filthy words fly. I wanted her to get off, wanted to be the one to take her to a higher place. I spread my fingers so that I was rubbing her on either side of her clit for a moment without touching her button directly. Then I used two fingers to start tapping out a rhythm on her clit—pat, pat, pat.

Giselle went nuts for this move. "Oh yes. Oh please." I started to tap her a little harder, and she whipped her head back and forth, clearly loving every single second. I used four fingers pressed together, and now I was practically spanking her clitoris and she was crying out my name over and over. I saw her reflection in the glass on one of the movie posters. She looked hot and untamed. I grasped her ponytail and pulled. She practically whinnied, and then looked at me over her shoulder once more. I saw light and fire in her eyes. She was right on the cusp. I watched the pleasure flicker all over her.

With one final mighty thrust I drove my cock inside her. She squeezed down hard on my dick as she came, and her whole body trembled. I let her ride out the full length of her climax before I got off, shooting my load deep inside her. Then I pulled out and waited to see what she'd do next. To my delight, she grabbed a blue blanket off the sofa and wrapped the two of us up. Then she reached for the remote, and with a guilty smile she said, "There's this Bogart movie on tonight. Do you want to watch a little with me?"

"You know the answer to that already," I told her, slipping one arm around her and settling back against the sofa to watch movie magic. We'd made our own magic already.

The Power of Three

EMILIE PARIS

A woman was on her hands and knees—one man behind her sliding his monster cock between her thighs, another man in front of her, feeding her the head of his dick. The girl handled the attention effortlessly. She basked in the attention of her two handsome lovers.

At least, she did in my drawings.

I sat dejectedly in the last meeting of the day—the last long-winded, boring-ass meeting in a day of long-winded, boring-ass meetings. To entertain myself, I drew dirty pictures in the margins and footers of the handouts I'd collected.

If I'd had a flask, I would have made my own drinking game. One swallow of whiskey for every time the speaker said, "Collaboration." It wasn't his fault. The speech was on enhancing corporate cooperation—and there are only so many ways to say that phrase. Still, my head throbbed. When the speaker told us to envision the parts of the company as three legs in a tri-legged stool, I let out an audible sigh of disgust. Immediately, heads turned to look at me, and I pretended to be yawning—which wasn't much better. I was supposed to look peppy and interested, not bored to tears.

To keep myself awake, I returned to the filthy fucking pictures I'd been penning on the edges of my papers.

"Nice," said a voice behind me.

I closed my binder quickly and peeked over my shoulder. William, the cutest of the cute boys from sales sat behind me on the left.

"I liked the one on the previous page better," he said.

I pretended not to know what he was talking about. Then a voice from my other side chimed in. "I agree," said the second man. "That sketch was spectacularly dirty."

I knew that voice. I looked over my right shoulder and saw Tim—the hot number-wizard from accounting.

Oh god. Oh god. Oh god. Why had I not covered my scribbles? Why had I zoned out? I'd thought there was no one in the row behind me. At a pause between the dull three-legged stool speaker and the next, a chirpy blonde woman who seemed to be doing her best impersonation of a human parakeet, the two men moved to either side of me.

"These speeches couldn't be more tedious if they tried," Will said.

"But this"—Tim opened my binder and pointed to one of the drawings—"*This* looks interesting."

It had been a while since I'd last had sex. My mind had gone to

7

that place where fantasies took over almost every waking moment. The drawings I'd made in the margins were like dirty diagrams for three-way encounters. The one Tim was pointing to showed a girl on her back with one man between her legs—and the other man behind the first. I turned as crimson as Will's tie.

"Are you staying for the cocktail meet-and-greet?" Will asked me conversationally.

I stammered nonsense words.

"Why don't we ditch?" suggested Tim. We all agreed that was best.

Quietly, we made our exit from the conference room while the parakeet pointed to a list of figures on the screen. The line on the chart, at least, was going up. I knew two other things that would be on the rise soon, as well.

Instead of driving to any one of our homes, Will checked us into the hotel where the lectures were being held. The fact that there were three of us—and that none of us had any luggage—wasn't commented upon by the clerk. In the elevator, things got heated right away. Will started to unbutton my blouse. Tim got behind me and lifted my skirt. I closed my eyes and basked in the attention of the two men. When Will had my shirt open, he pulled down the cups of my black satin bra and began to kiss my nipples—first one, then the other. I cried out at the feeling of his wet mouth on my flushed skin. I could feel my pussy clenching. So could Tim, who had slid his fingers into my panties from behind and was sinuously thrusting two digits into my pussy. He seemed to be working in time with the sucking of Will's mouth—and I had a second to think about the power of cooperation before I was wracked with giddy giggles.

The bell of the elevator alerted us to the fact that we'd arrived.

We tripped over ourselves to get to the room, with me holding my blouse closed and Tim doing his best to make me lower my hands. What if someone walked by us? What if someone spotted our debauchery? Actually, those possibilities only made me more turned on.

As soon as the door was open, we rushed into the room. There was no pausing at the minibar. We didn't even bother to close the blinds. With Tim's help, I stripped off my outfit. Will took off his own clothes, and he and I began to make out. I'd admired him ever since I'd joined the company, but I'd never thought anything like this would ever happen. I assumed that everyone at the firm was as stuffy as the firm itself.

Tim positioned me on the bed, and then the boys joined me. I realized that we were making my dirty margin art come to life. Will got in front of me, and I began to blow him. I sucked and slurped at his rod while Tim stood behind me and gripped my hips. I had a moment to suck in a deep breath before Tim speared me. "Oh fuck," I whimpered, panting before I started working Will with my mouth again.

Right as I was on the verge of coming, the boys switched spots. They must have created some signal between them, because I wasn't expecting the swap. Then I was sucking Tim and being fucked by Will. I started moaning at the pleasure, and I guess the vibrations of my utterances took Tim past his limits. He came down my throat in a river, and I swallowed every drop.

Will held on. He kept fucking me at a slow, steady pace, and when Tim had caught his breath, he slipped under my body and began to lick my clit. I sussed out the fact that he was doing more than that, lapping at the juncture where Will and I connected. Will made a grunting sound deep in his throat, and I imagined that Tim was lapping at his friend's balls. That thought, combined with the sporadic attention Tim paid to my clit, took me through the ring of fire. I came in what felt like a crescendo—a burst of sound all around me that I didn't recognize immediately had come from my mouth. I was moaning loud enough for Tim to move around and muffle my noises with his cock again.

Thank god I had something to keep me busy. Even as I was still creaming, I sucked him again, thinking that he would come in my mouth as an encore. I was surprised when he didn't. I was even more surprised when he got off the bed, his hand pumping his cock. I turned to look in the mirror, and I realized he was getting behind Will. We became a chain, a train, Tim fucking Will, who was fucking me. The climaxes this time felt like a scientific reaction—one setting off the next setting off the last.

I had never felt like that before. I wasn't merely used up. I was demolished by pleasure. We came apart and lay there on the bed, overlapping and breathless.

"Just look what can happen when we collaborate," Tim said, his mouth all shiny with my juices. Will bent forward to lick Tim's lips clean, and I realized I'd never look at mandatory teamwork in the same way again.

Spank You Later

Alison Tyler

The text was simple enough. The words on the screen read: *Spank you later.*

I wondered for a moment if autocorrect had gotten the best of Daniel's smartphone. But there was no way "see" had been turned to "spank." And he wouldn't have been "thanking" me for anything that I could think of. No, the text definitely read: *Spank you later.* I crossed my legs and shifted on my seat. Damn. I'd been focused on work, and now I couldn't think straight. I wrote him back:

What's that supposed to mean?

His response was almost instantaneous: *What do you think it means?*

I sat there staring in silence. Then I went outside with my phone and called Dan. He answered with a normal hello. He didn't seem to find anything odd about the text he'd sent.

"Daniel…" I said. I didn't want to have to ask. I wanted him to explain himself.

I could hear the warmth in his voice. He said, "Come to my house tonight. Wear a skirt. I'll clear up everything then."

I did exactly what he said. After work, I stripped out of my professional attire and chose a pretty, flirty mini. I wore a pair of thigh-high stockings, fixed my hair and makeup, and spritzed on my favorite perfume. Feeling fluttery to my very core, I drove to my boyfriend's house. During the whole drive, I lost myself in thoughts of being spanked. By the time Daniel opened his door for me, I was awash in trembles. How had he known? That was my biggest query. How had he figured out that the spanking letters in *Penthouse Variations* were the ones that always made me wet? That I kept my treasured editions tucked under my mattress.

That's exactly what had done me in. Daniel said, "Remember when I spent the night at your place a few weeks ago, and I helped you strip the bed?"

Oh, for the love of god. He'd found my back issues.

"While you were in the shower, I read the pages you'd marked. Every time I've come over, I've read a little more. I kept waiting for you to make the move, to tell me what you wanted. Then I got tired of waiting. Tonight, I thought we might bring one of those scenes to life."

I swallowed hard. I shifted from one foot to the other. I waited for Daniel's instruction.

"Now, if I remember correctly, the situations you seem most drawn to are the ones where the man bends the lady over his lap. Is that correct?"

I nodded.

"You'll answer when I ask you a question," he said, but he winked at me to soften the statement.

"Yes, Daniel."

Immediately, he bent me over—as if he'd been putting girl-friends into proper spanking position for years. I found myself staring down at the floor, my long hair cascading toward the polished hard-wood. I contemplated the fact that I'd read about this type of scenario often enough, but I'd never found myself upended before.

"Let me know if I'm doing this right," Daniel said wryly, and he slowly lifted my skirt in the back. I could feel that he was hard, and that gave me a jolt of pleasure. As turned on as I was, it seemed that Daniel was at least equally so. When he had my skirt bunched up at the waist, he let one big hand rest on my panty-clad ass. "I think we should start slowly for the first time," Daniel said. "I'll give you ten. Then we can pause and see how you're feeling."

He started right away, spanking me with gusto, and he counted the blows out loud, ticking them off from one to ten. The spanking passed in a blur of bliss. All of my fantasies came true in those few seconds. But then the night got even better. When he was finished, I was breathless and wetter than I'd ever been. Daniel discovered this himself when he pulled down my panties and let his fingertips wander along the juicy split of my slick pussy lips.

"See, now that's a shame," Daniel said.

"What is?" I managed to whisper.

"Well, here I am spanking you, and you've gotten all kinds of turned on. I thought a punishment was supposed to mean something."

"It did," I babbled uselessly, focused on the way my hot bottom felt. "It did mean something."

He laughed. "Apparently, it means you got turned on. We'll have to try something a little more serious." Suddenly, he was spanking me on my bare asscheeks, and a whole new world of intoxication erupted inside me. Yes, I'd been a fan of spanking tales for years, but the reality of having my own *tail* spanked was something both erotic and beautiful.

Daniel's hand smacked back and forth—first on my left cheek, then my right, and then back again. He didn't seem as cautious as he'd been at first, and my ass quickly took on a powerful, tingling sensation. That didn't stop me from squirming my hips and grinding against his lap. My pussy felt as much on fire as my ass—but different—liquid fire, molten lava. I was all heated up inside. Daniel seemed to understand. He parted my thighs so that his fingertips could deliver lighter taps between. When he touched my clit, I cried out. When he rubbed that throbbing button, I climaxed in a tumultuous rush. I couldn't remember ever coming like that before. The thrilling heat of my first spanking, combined with the way Daniel rotated his fingers on my clitoris, had me whimpering with pleasure across his lap.

As soon as the orgasm had crested, Daniel slid me over onto the mattress. He stood behind me and admired his handiwork. I looked over my shoulder at him as he said, "You have the most amazing ass. And it's never looked as gorgeous as right now. Your rear end was simply made to be spanked." He manhandled the smarting globes, commenting the whole time on how ripe and red they looked. "Like cherries," he said. "I could bite one."

To my delight, he did, bending to nip at my derriere. I squealed and rubbed at the love bite.

"Did you like your first spanking?" Daniel asked as he took his clothes off and joined me on the bed.

"Oh, yes."

"Then tell me. Tell me everything." As he spoke, he slid his cock inside me. I closed my eyes and let myself bask in the lusciousness of Daniel fucking me. Each thrust forward reminded me of the way his palm had felt on my bottom, how sexy I'd felt when he'd pulled down my panties. "Tell me," Daniel said, and I could hear the yearning in his voice.

"I loved feeling your cock against me," I told him, "pressing up against me while your hand flashed over and over on my ass. It hurt," I continued, "but the hurt was swallowed up instantly by something else. Something better." I found talking difficult based on the fucking Daniel was giving me. But I sensed he wanted me to keep describing the feelings, so I did my best.

"I can't wait for you to spank me with other items," I said. "Your belt. A paddle. A wooden spoon." All the stories I'd read before came bubbling to life in my mind. I could imagine Daniel making every last one of my fantasies come true. "I can't fucking wait," I gushed.

Daniel groaned. I was clearly getting to him.

"When you come, shoot all over my ass," I begged him. He helped me to climax one more time, and then he did what I asked, shooting all over my hot bottom, then rubbing the sticky juices into my burning skin.

We collapsed together on the bed, both of us mildly shocked by what we'd done—but definitely excited. We'd reached a new level in our relationship, and it was all thanks to my collection of dirty stories.

Hot Stuff

Priscilla Lawrence

Bonnie's sparkling ass was what caught my attention first. I know so many people claim their partner's eyes or smile or musical laugh did them in. But for me—it was her ass. I'd been sitting at a corner table in my favorite café on campus when she strode to the counter and ordered a Shot in the Dark. That's my drink, too, and I glanced up to see who'd placed the order.

Her ass was what I saw first—dark denim jeans, to be specific, the pockets emblazoned with rhinestones that glittered whenever she moved. And she moved a lot. She leaned on her toes to snag a packet of raw sugar. She bent way over to grab her wallet out of the purse she'd dropped at her side. She was in motion for the entire order, it seemed, and I sat captivated by the disco-like pattern on her back pockets.

Complementing the bejeweled behind was a bright sunny T-shirt and cork-heeled sandals. Her long blonde hair cascaded loose and shiny past her shoulders.

I recognized her from one of my art history lectures, but I'd never seen her standing. Now that I caught the full fabulousness of her physique, I couldn't bear the thought of her walking out of the café and out of my life, or at least out of my morning. As she fastened the cap on her to-go cup, I got behind her—a little too close behind her. She spun to leave, and then she gasped, "Oh, I'm sorry," as if it were her fault, when really *I'd* stepped into *her* space.

"I'd like to take a shot in the dark," I said quickly, "and see if you'd like to have your coffee with me."

She looked me up and down. I saw a glimmer of recognition in her blue eyes. So maybe she'd noticed me, too. I felt the heat between us. If nobody had been around us, I would have kissed her. But I gripped one of her hands in mine and squeezed.

"To go?" she asked, and there was the husky whisper of promised sex in her voice. I hurried to grab my book and my own cup of joe. We strolled to her apartment, close by campus, exchanging names and then gossiping about different professors we'd had in common, classes we liked and disliked. I kept stealing surreptitious—or so I thought—glances at her ass. Until she said, "Wait until we get upstairs. Then you can see the whole package." Maybe I wasn't so surreptitious after all.

In her sunlit apartment, we set down the coffees and our bags and then, before any awkwardness could set in, she was undressing. I leaned against the wall and watched her. She slipped off her yellow V-neck, her sandals, and then she started to work on those painted-on jeans. I couldn't stand the suspense. I came over and helped her, pulling them down myself and going on my knees at the same time. I pressed her up against the arm of her sofa and set my mouth against the front of her panties. These were a lighter yellow than her T-shirt and nearly sheer. I licked her through the fabric and she sighed, letting me know I was on the right track to her pleasure stop.

"I've wanted you to do this since the start of the semester," she said, placing her hands on my shoulders as I sucked hard on the fabric covering her pussy.

"Really?" I asked breathlessly, breaking from her only long enough to slide her panties down.

"I didn't know if you'd noticed me," she said. "I always tried to sit where I could see you and the professor."

"You can see me now," I told her, "and that turns me on." I loved feeling her eyes on me while I worked her. Now I could suck on her clit without the hindrance of the panties. I held her shaved nether lips open as I tongued her button. She moaned and arched for me, lifting herself onto the arm of the sofa and spreading her thighs as wide as they would go.

I brought one hand into play, inserting my pointer into her pussy as I kept working her clit. She moaned and shivered as I finger-fucked her, and then she let out that sexy gasp again as I used the wet tip of my finger to trace all around her snug asshole. Had I thought her ass was adorable in those jeans? Naked, her rear end was even more of a delight. When I slid my finger into her rear hole, she came, her muscles clutching my digit in tight spasms while her pussy seemed to flutter under my tongue. I kept at her until she moved out of my reach, undone by the sensations. I sat back on my haunches, waiting to see what would happen next—and what happened was this:

She led me to her tiny bedroom and said, "Take off your clothes." I hurried to obey while she rummaged in a drawer of her dresser. I was naked when she approached with a two-headed dildo and a bottle of lube. "I took a shot in the dark," she said, playing with my opening gambit, "when I bought this. I hoped I'd have someone to try it out with before too long. And now I do."

She slid one end of the dildo into her pussy, lubed up the other end and lay down on the bed. I joined her, with my pussy close to hers, and I slid the free end of the toy into my own snatch. Then we were connected. It only took us a few seconds to figure out a good rhythm of rocking back and forth so that the dildo was our connecting rod and the waves of intensity were almost overwhelming. She kept one hand on the toy, and I felt more or less of the rod going inside me as we seesawed together.

"That feels so good," I heard myself saying. I hadn't even known I was going to speak. She made a low cooing sound of pleasure.

I started to frig my own clit while squeezing the dildo, and I realized in a rush that I was going to come—and I did so, loudly, crying out her name. "Bonnie, oh fuck. Bonnie!" She came a beat after me, whimpering, "Priscilla," as she tossed her head and let those waves of hair fly.

We very gently parted, extracting the toy in tandem and then falling into each other in a sticky embrace. But I was far from done. Her ass had won my attention at the start. Now I needed to bestow upon those rounded curves the satisfaction they deserved. I rolled her over and began to lick and kiss my way up one mound of flesh and down to the valley. Bonnie held still, seeming to know where I was going. I parted her rear cheeks and began to kiss lightly between them.

She grabbed a pillow and placed it under her hips, raising her body up to help me.

With slow decadence, I started to rim her. I used my tongue to tease and tickle, and then I brought my hand under her body to softly stroke her clit. The combination of tactics had Bonnie on the verge quickly. I sealed my mouth to her rosebud and licked while pinching her clit in a pulse-like beat. That technique took Bonnie over the edge, and she came in a series of violent shudders that rocked the whole bed.

I am so glad I decided to take my studies to the café. I found more than history about a long-dead empire. I found my new girlfriend.

Behind the Curtain

BELLA DEAN

Rory does trade shows for his water filtration company. He's always the man in charge, and it's always a one-man job.

Rory's also extremely neat, and when he assembles his show setup, he includes a black curtain behind his booth that's printed with the company's logo. The fabric conceals his boxes and suitcases and such. The curtain is long enough to brush the floor, and it's totally opaque. In other words, it's perfect.

I often accompany him on his trips. Usually, I sightsee and wander the show floor or hit the local pubs and restaurants while I wait for him to be finished with his work. But for certain shows, the slow ones, he'll whisper in my ear, "Come back at eleven. I'll take a break."

His last show was one of those slow ones. So at eleven I tottered in on sexy heels, wearing a knee-length black sheath dress. My long dark hair was ironed straight, my lips slicked red. When I caught sight of him, my heart started to pound. When he grinned at me across the sparse crowd, my pussy got wet inside my panties.

"There she is," he said softly when I arrived. He rummaged under the table and found a sign that read BACK IN 15 and put it on the table, front and center.

I chewed my lip softly, my nervous habit betraying my arousal.

During these lulls, I like to suck his cock behind his signature black curtain. It fulfills his needs and mine, because while I'm sucking him, I'm wondering if we'll get caught, which turns me on. Then I usually spend the remainder of the day in a happy stupor, waiting for him to be done so he can bring me to our room and fuck me.

"Here I am," I whispered, slipping behind the table, wandering as nonchalantly as I could behind the curtain. The fabric fell down to brush the floor once more, and there I was, invisible and cloaked to passersby.

A moment later Rory appeared, carefully brushing the curtain back into place. He went right for his button and zipper even as he said softly, "On your knees."

I dropped to my knees obligingly, my pussy clenching tight at his demanding words. I shivered in my sexy dress, on my already tender knees, waiting.

He stepped toward me, his cock free and his hand stroking. He flashed another wolfish grin and said, "My god, you look gorgeous today. Let's see what you can do with that pretty mouth. And then..." He took another step closer to me, and I was almost breathless. "If you're really good, I'll take care of you tonight. Just like you need."

I nodded. Yes. Just like I needed. But the truth was, I needed this as much as what he'd do to me later. I needed to see the effect my mouth would have on him. To see how his face took on a peaceful but cautious look, to feel his come pumping across my tongue, my lips... my chin.

I smiled, reaching for him, but he shook his head. "No, no," he tsked. "Hands down."

I put my hands at my sides, and then went one step further and put my hands behind my back, clasping one wrist with the opposite hand.

He was close to me now. Close. I could smell soap and arousal on him. He ran the head of his cock along my lower lip, and when he was dead center, he tapped my lip a few times with his shaft. I shut my eyes and let my tongue dart out to taste him. The moment we connected, he made a noise in his throat.

Excitement unfurled in me, sudden and delightful. I clenched my internal muscles just to feel that delicious pressure. Then I wrapped my lips around his cock and moved forward slowly, sucking him in as wetly as I could.

"Only your mouth, baby. No hands. Keep them back there. Keep them out of this."

I nodded my understanding even as I pressed forward, taking him into my mouth and then my throat.

"Mmm, nice," he said.

He gripped the sides of my head and held me as he thrust forward eagerly to fill my mouth. His strokes were short and brutal, stealing my breath and bringing tears to my eyes.

"Good, good..." he sighed, and my cunt grew even more drenched.

I released a moan, pushing myself to my limits. I sucked harder, taking him deeper as my eyes watered and my shoulders trembled from holding myself just so.

He pulled free of my mouth, and I gasped. Then, tracing my lips with his cockhead as if applying lip gloss, he watched the play of his dick over my bright red lips.

"I like your lipstick," he said.

I darted my tongue out to tease him. He tasted richer now that he was fully aroused. It was perfect.

Someone beyond the curtain said, "Sign says back in fifteen. Wait or go?"

Another voice answered, "Wait."

I groaned so softly I barely heard it, but he chuckled. "I guess we have visitors. Go ahead, then. Lift that dress. Get off with me. This time I'd like you to. I want to see."

He pushed his cock back in, forcing it along my tongue, past my teeth, filling my mouth. I inhaled deeply again and did as I was told. I hiked up my dress around my hips and pulled my panties to the side. Then I began to tease my clitoris before sliding a finger inside my wet cunt.

"That's it," he said. His voice was growing wispier. He was close, and that alone covered my skin with goose bumps.

He held the side of my head, blocking out much of my sound, and fucked my mouth.

I drove a second finger into my pussy and ground my palm against my clitoris. The penetration and pressure had me close to coming within moments.

"I'll tell you when you can. You hear me? Not before. Do not come before me."

I nodded—still licking, still sucking. The tip of his cock brushed the back of my throat, and I nearly gagged but didn't. My cheeks ached from sucking, my tongue tired from swishing and looping and whirling.

"Jesus," he said. "Best cocksucker ever. My wife, ladies and gentlemen."

He began to thrust hard into my mouth, taking over. I relaxed a tad and let him use me. Let him set the pace.

His lips pressed together, and his eyes slammed shut. After a minute, Rory moaned. "Now!"

My exploring fingers, which had never stopped their mission, triggered my G-spot and I came, gasping around his cock. I tried to keep my sounds low and soft. I climaxed on my knees as he spilled into my mouth, a fine line of cream rolling down my chin as I continued to lap at him.

He stepped away quickly, putting himself back in order as fast as he could. Then he held out a hand to help me up. When I started to arrange myself to be presentable, he shook his head. Then he righted my panties, tugged my dress down, took a tissue from his pocket and wiped my lips.

Rory kissed me and winked. "Put more lipstick on and fix your hair. I'll meet you back at the hotel room at six."

I nodded, sex-drunk.

"And sweetheart, you better be ready. Oh, the things I plan to do to you…"

Then he disappeared to the other side of his magical black curtain, and I heard him exclaim heartily, "Gentlemen! Thank you for waiting!"

Deep Desires

CHRISTOPHER MONROE

My wife, Donna, loves me more than anything. I have felt the warmth of her adoration for the past twelve years. This is why she fucked her coworker David last night. I'd finally confessed to my darling wife that more than anything else in the entire world, I wanted to see her screw another man.

I have to say, she took the news better than I would have expected.

We sat there in the living room, on our blush-pink sofa, and Donna simply smiled at me and said, "When?"

"What do you mean when?" I asked her, startled.

"When do you want to see me fuck another man?" she asked in her calm, matter-of-fact way.

"You mean you will?" I babbled. "Just like that?" My hand shook when I set my wineglass back on the coffee table.

Donna caught the glass and laughed at my reaction. "Of course," she said. "If that's something you'd like to see, I'd be more than happy to make your fantasy a reality."

I couldn't believe it. I don't know what I'd expected, honestly. I'd felt telling her was the important part, but I'd had no idea how she might react to my confession. This was such startlingly good news I could hardly fathom my luck. This was also beyond my expertise, actually. I had no clue how to answer her next question either, which was simply: "Do you have someone in mind?"

"Well, I don't know," I said. "I've never gotten that far."

Donna kissed me, and she stroked me through my slacks. I was dangerously erect. If she pulled out my cock and merely kissed the tip, I would have gone off on her lips. "Then leave it up to me," she said. "You come home tomorrow, right on time, and I'll make your wickedest dreams come true."

We fucked like porn stars after that. I had her every which way, never even making it to the bedroom. The whole time, I thought of who she might do, how she might look.

Needless to say, I hardly managed to get anything done at work the following day. I tried. I turned on my computer. I clicked on files. I even made a phone call or two. But all I could think about was Donna, my gorgeous dreamy wife, fucking someone else—someone of her choosing—someone while I watched.

When I got home, there was Donna's little red convertible in the driveway, and a big pickup truck was nestled right behind it, as if trying to fuck the bumper. I wracked my brain to remember if I'd ever seen that truck before. It looked familiar, but there are a lot of trucks in town. I walked to the door, and I could already hear Donna's laughter before I slid my key in the lock. I entered but didn't call out hello or say anything. Donna had given me no instructions, so I wasn't sure if I was supposed to be loud to announce my entrance, or stealthy.

I followed the sighs and moans to the master bedroom. There was Donna, and with her was David, who I recognized immediately from office functions. He was in charge of the warehouse where Donna works, and he had the muscles of a man who knows how to move merchandise, even if he's moved his way up to management. Now, he was moving Donna. They were both naked, and she was straddling him while he jostled her up and down, his big hands tight around her slim waist.

The couple was busy, but they looked up when I walked in.

"Hi, honey," Donna said, as if every day of the week I walk in to catch her fucking a hunky stud.

"Hi, Christopher," said David, and he winked at me. Winked!

"I told David that you had this fantasy," Donna purred, "and he was a hundred percent down for helping you out. So have a seat." She indicated the leather armchair near the bed. I sat down and stared. My cock was so hard, I couldn't keep my hands off myself. I slowly started to stroke my dick through my pants while David returned to bouncing my wife.

All my fantasies put together paled in comparison to how sexy this couple looked. He was so well built that I could tell his hobby was working out. Donna fit well with him, her slender body moving up and down his formidable dick. Suddenly, I needed to see that part. I needed to see the place where they were joined. I quietly moved closer to the bed. The couple didn't pay me any attention. I got into a position that allowed me to see his greasy cock sliding in and out of her wet hole.

That was the prettiest sight I'd ever seen: Donna's shaved puss being speared by his massive manhood. They changed positions then, David deciding to go missionary with my wife. He spread her out on the bed, and then he began to thrust his cock deep inside her. Donna wrapped her long, lean legs around his body, pulling him into her. As she did, she started to talk. "Dave, you're so big. Fuck me harder, baby. Fuck me harder."

David seemed to take direction well. He kept slamming his body against Donna's over and over, and then she changed tactics. She started talking to me instead of him. "After he shoots, Christopher, then it will be your turn. I'll have his warm, wet come deep inside me, and you'll be able to feel his jism all over your dick."

Donna had never talked like that in her life. At least, she hadn't talked to *me* like that. I couldn't believe the words she was saying. I thought I might rocket off right then in my pants, but thankfully the words seemed to have worked their magic on David, who announced his orgasm with a mighty moan.

He pulled out and moved over on the bed, apparently in no need to rush out the door. I didn't care. All that mattered to me at that moment was fucking Donna. I stripped out of my clothes faster than I ever had before, and I got onto the bed with my beauty. In the same position, I started to fuck her, and I made sure to toggle her clit while I worked her. I wanted us to get off together when we reached our limits.

I found that I actually liked being watched by David. That was surprising to me. I had only ever fantasized about watching my wife—I had never thought about being watched! Then he did something completely unexpected. He started talking.

"Fuck her hard, man," David said. "Fuck her like the bad girl she is. And then you know what?" I looked over at him. He was leaning against our headboard, lazily stroking his massive meat. "Then we can take turns eating out her wet cunt."

That sent Donna into the stratosphere. I felt her climax, her inner muscles squeezing and releasing me repeatedly. I came one beat later, filling her up the way David had. I looked at her to see if she was willing to do what her new lover had suggested. Donna kissed me and blushed, and I could tell that she was more than willing.

David surprised me by taking the first turn. He got between Donna's legs, and he licked and sucked her pussy. I knew he must have been tasting my semen mixed with her sweet nectar, but he didn't seem to have a problem with that. When he made her come, he moved aside, and I knew it was my turn. I overlapped two fingers to create a corkscrew, and I finger-fucked Donna while I slurped her pussy juices and tongued her swollen clit.

When Donna came on my tongue, I was so happy. I loved our new little triangle of pleasure, and as soon as we'd all caught our breath, I said so. David has promised to come over next Saturday, and this time he said he'll take the first turn watching, and I'll have the first turn licking out sweet Donna's honeypot.

One thing I know for sure—our sex life will never be the same again.

Corporate Affairs

Sadie Reynolds

Ladd and I aren't swanky party people. We're more the beer-and-burger type. But occasionally he has an event from work he can't miss. Which means I can't miss it, either. The last time his company held an award ceremony, my husband informed me that there was no way we could escape the event.

"Can't be avoided," he said, looking through his closet to see what might be suitable to wear.

I was pillaging my closet, feeling a little desperate, when he stuck his head in and said, "I should tell you that there are rumors about the VP and his wife."

I froze. "Rumors?"

"Yeah." He waggled his eyebrows in a comical way and stage-whispered, "Sexual rumors."

My fear was swiftly displaced by excitement. "As in?"

"They like to swap."

My stomach dropped as if I were on an airborne plane. "What does he look like?"

He shrugged. "Handsome. Your type."

"And her?"

"Gorgeous." This time I got a playful wink. "Not nearly as gorgeous as my wife, but she'll do in a pinch."

I laughed. She was probably a knockout. I abandoned my closet and grabbed him by the front of his pale blue button-down shirt. "Are you thinking...?"

When he pushed his hands into my plaid leggings and slipped a finger into my cunt, I knew he was definitely thinking what I was thinking. And then he proceeded to prove it to me by fucking me senseless.

The night of the party came faster than I had expected considering we had an agenda. I put on my nicest little black dress, some sling-back sandals and my pearls that hung down my back, swinging in the space left by the low-cut, open-backed dress.

"Spectacular," Ladd said, gathering me in his arms. "I think we might have a good night."

"You think?" I asked, hopeful.

"I do."

The party was a crowd of the rich and elegant. The food was off the charts, the music subdued but lively at the same time. When Ladd waved me over to introduce me to the VP and his wife, my hands began to shake.

"Sweetheart, this is Keven, our VP, and his wife, Marie."

I shook hands and felt my heart jolt a little when the missus gave my hand an extra squeeze. "So nice to meet you. Your husband was just saying wonderful things about you."

I swallowed hard as we made chitchat. My mind was off and running as I studied Keven, who was tall and broad, with dark-brown hair and warm brown eyes. I had to focus my attention on not letting my gaze wander to his crotch. I saw Ladd give a small smile because he could read my mind.

The party carried on, and right around the point where I was more than ready to go, Ladd came over and whispered, "Keven and Marie want to know if we'd like to come back to their house for a nightcap."

"And you said?"

"Really, doll?" he asked, patting my ass lightly. "Is that an actual question?"

So, of course, we went.

Once in their house—which was honestly more of a mansion—Marie turned to me. "When Keven and I swap, we like to be in the same room. Would that be a problem?"

I blinked. She was so direct and soft-spoken; I was slightly stunned.

"Not at all," Ladd interjected. "If anything, it adds to the experience."

"I agree," she said, smiling.

That was the extent of the pre-fucking talk. Keven came toward me and touched the back of my dress. "May I?"

I nodded, and he began to pull my dress off slowly. I was braless, but he made quick, sensual work of removing my panties and my hose. He dropped down on his knees to drag his tongue along my belly, and I quivered. For Ladd, Marie was the aggressor. A rush of fluid escaped me as I watched her lower his pants and pull his cock free of his briefs. She hummed softy as if pleased.

Just then, Keven pushed his hands up my inner thighs and set his mouth to my pussy. I watched, mesmerized, as Marie knelt and took Ladd into her mouth. She sucked him deeply, working a hand up beneath her lovely navy-blue shift dress.

And then I was lost in what Keven was doing with his mouth. It only took him a minute or two to make me come. I grabbed his short, neat hair and pressed my pussy to his mouth as I climaxed. I was loud and saw our spouses glance up and smile. Ladd was removing Marie's dress when Keven turned me on my hands and knees. I heard him getting undressed. Then the snap of a condom hit my ears and my nipples spiked from the sound. From the knowledge of what was soon to come.

He gripped my hips and ran his sheathed cock along my asscrack, pausing briefly at my anus before traveling down and nudging the tip of his cock inside me. I heard Ladd grunt softly, a sound I knew to be pleasure, and I followed it with a moan. Hearing him that way only served to turn me on more.

Keven thrust deep, and my G-spot flooded me with pleasure. Keven's cock was thicker than Ladd's and seemed to touch places that had gone unnoticed for a long time. My new lover wound his hand in my hair and tugged hard enough to send a thrill skittering through me. "Touch yourself for me. Come again. I want to feel you around my cock."

I shuddered as I moved my hand to obey. The dirty talk was

only going to set me off faster. I touched my clit with trembling fingers, spreading my own juices around as lubricant.

His rhythm picked up, his hand in my hair gripping firmly, the one clutching my hip just rough enough to force my pleasure higher.

"God, yes," I said softly.

I heard Ladd echo me and wondered what Marie was doing to him. With him. For him. But hearing and not seeing was a lovely experience. It let me focus on the rush of pleasure that coursed through me. I found myself slamming back to take Keven's thick cock. I rubbed my clit hard, showing myself no mercy with the almost overwhelming stimulation.

Keven worked a finger into my ass, and I whimpered, letting my head hang down and my body surge back to meet him.

"Christ. Right like that," he said, raspy and rough.

I squeezed my cunt, and when I heard Marie let out a long, soft cry I came. The sound of the other couple fucking set me off unexpectedly.

"What a good girl Ladd has," Keven said, and I damn near came again.

I heard Ladd grunt and sigh the way he does right before he climaxes. I rubbed and stroked my clitoris furiously, wanting so badly to come one more time. I bit my lip and shut my eyes, and when I heard him come, I slammed back against Keven. He wasn't immune to the sounds either. He said, "Christ," again softly and then drove into me for one final thrust. He went stiff, cried out, and that was all I needed for my third and final orgasm.

My body trembled, and my hair swayed around my face. I stayed that way for a moment, frozen on my hands and knees as my muscles worked their way up to moving again. I was boneless, satiated. Drunk on pleasure.

When I turned, Marie looked very pleased and Ladd looked pretty happy. He curled a finger at me, and I went to him, kissing him deeply.

Marie, still nude, went to pour our drinks. Her cheeks were rosy, her hair tousled. "You know," she said, handing out crystal glasses of whiskey. "We're going on a trip next week. Nude beaches, sun, sand, fun. We love traveling companions. Think you'd be interested?"

I looked at Ladd, excited for the prospect of a compatible couple and an exotic location.

He chuckled. "I don't know. I'd have to check into getting off work."

Keven, the VP, laughed, and then winked at me. "Don't worry, Ladd. I think I can help you out with that."

Butterfingers

Victoria Neilson

Chet is a big lumbering man. He's clumsy, too, except for when he isn't. He can be the most delicate-handed man in the world when working with watches and clocks, which is what he does for a living. His specialty is antique grandfather clocks. But when he's just moving through his everyday life, he can be like a bull in a china shop.

People are often surprised by our age difference. I'm fourteen years older than him. Fifty-two to his thirty-eight. Chet always jokes that he got a two-for-one deal: a wife and a mother figure for the price of one.

A few weeks ago, while helping me with chores, he broke my vacuum by dropping it. The machine was a high-priced, fancy number that required no bag and was battery-charged. It wasn't cheap, and to ing in three chunks at the foot of the steps took my breath away.

He stopped midway down the flight of stairs, looking shame-faced. "Sorry, baby. Sorry. It just…slipped out of my grasp."

I stared at him. Seeing how upset he was, I felt a little bad, but I was also a little mad. I shook my head. "Are you serious? You dropped it?"

He hung his head and nodded, saying nothing.

Rage danced with pity inside me, and I didn't quite know what to do with myself—until he shifted his big body in a certain way that made me think of when we were fucking. When we were *playing*. And suddenly I knew how to salvage at least something from this situation.

"Get down here!" I pointed my finger to the hardwood floor in front of my stomping foot.

His green eyes flew wide, and a look that was part terror and part excitement swept over his face. He was flustered, and two large red spots appeared on his cheeks. I almost smiled but kept my mirth to myself.

Chet moved slowly, the way a cowed dog would, and I snapped my fingers. "Move it. Today, Chet."

"Yes, Ma'am," he muttered.

I inhaled deeply as if tasting the air. Ah, words to cherish. *Yes, Ma'am.*

"Pants off. Briefs off. On your knees—now."

I let all the anger from seeing my lovely fancy vacuum demol-ished seep into my tone. There was no room for argument, and punish-ment was imminent.

He slowly took off his pants and underwear, pausing to take off his socks, too, because he knows I can't stand when he leaves them on.

Then he knelt in front of me.

I glanced around the living room and found what I was after. "Now, it seems you have a hard time holding on to things. Things that cost a lot of money. So you're going to practice holding on to something for me. No matter what happens," I barked.

I went to the corner and grabbed the whisk broom I'd propped there the night before. "Arms over your head," I said. His arms shot up instantly, and again I had to stifle a smile. I put the broom into his hands so that he was holding it horizontally. "Don't drop it," I said, sarcasm dripping from my tongue. "Because it's the only thing we have to clean the floor at the moment."

I saw his jaw clench, and he held the broom, straight-armed and rigid.

I walked in slow circles around him, building his anticipation and his dread. "You know I have to punish you. I saved forever for that goddamn vacuum."

I went to our bedroom and found my favorite leather paddle, the one with the word SLUT spelled out across the business end. I love to use it while telling him he's my little slut. Those words make him rock hard, and he delivers the most delicious oral sex when I scold him that way.

I returned to him with the paddle in hand and said, "Don't you dare drop that broom. Don't you dare let your arms sag. You stay exactly as you are and don't fuck it up."

Then I swatted his right buttock three times in rapid succession. He whimpered and his arms wavered, but he stayed strong. I glanced around to the front of him and found his cock standing out like a divining rod. I returned to my work, delivering two hard whacks to his left cheek, and then for the third, I alternated to keep him off balance. I landed the final blow horizontally across them both. His ass was a lovely shade of red, his dick as hard as stone. I detected a fine tremor in his arms.

His face was flushed, and he was sweating. Perfect.

I got down on my knees behind him and whispered close to his ear. "Not even close to being done yet, big boy. Just so you know." I dragged the top of the paddle down his asscrack and watched him flinch. Then to make it all so much better and so much worse, I gave him a very brief reach around. I gripped his cock, jacked it once and let it go.

He sobbed.

I explored his ass again with the paddle before sliding it softly along his lower back. When I saw his muscles relax a bit, I went for it. I paddled him fast and hard along the very bottom of his asscheeks. Then down the backs of his thighs. When he was trembling and his skin was red, I dropped the paddle and studied his grip on the broom. It was solid.

"Very good," I murmured. I walked to face him and removed the broom from his death grip. He hardly seemed to want to let it go. "You did well. You deserve a treat."

I lifted up my long skirt, shucked my panties and pulled his head unceremoniously to my crotch. He was on me in an instant, knowing what I wanted—what I needed—from him. He sucked and licked, working his tongue into my cunt before going back to sweep it over my aching clit.

I yanked his hair and drove my hips forward, pinching my own nipple with my free hand for added stimulation. I writhed against his tongue, taking whatever he wasn't delivering, but for the most part, Chet was delivering everything. All his sorrow over having broken the vacuum, from disappointing me, he put into his work.

"I want your fingers in me," I announced. "Hurry!"

I was so close to coming that I felt my knees trembling. My chest hurt with the need to come. When he shoved his fingers inside me, long and thick, I gasped. I rocked against that hand, savoring the alternating gentle and not-so-gentle motions of his tongue.

He added a third finger, then he sucked my clitoris hard. Then he lapped at my nub repeatedly until I lost my resolve and came with a violent cry.

I stared down at him and felt better. About the vacuum and about everything. I nodded to Chet. "You may come on my feet, and then you'd better clean up your mess. And do a good job."

Then I gave him what he needed—standing there stern and disapproving while he furiously jerked off, tugging so hard I marveled at the sight. When he spilled his seed across my feet, he made a sound from deep in his chest that turned me on all over again. My arousal flared fresh and sudden.

I patted his head. "Good boy," I said. "Now clean up. I think I have a few more things I want you to do for me today. We can worry about the vacuum later."

Cooking Up Kink

SOMMER MARSDEN

We were supposed to be cleaning the house out a few weeks ago. The plan was to gather everything we didn't use and donate it to charity. Better karma, cleaner house. The kitchen was the hardest because Dean is the kind of man who loves to cook and loves gadgets. We owned almost everything you can imagine for the kitchen marked AS SEEN ON TV.

I pulled out a long tool with a many-stranded silicone head. It was almost as big as a large paintbrush but not quite. I waved it at him. "What the hell is this?"

"It's a baster," he said. "Or a grill mop. Or whatever you call it."

"You own the thing, and you don't know what to call it?"

"It came with something."

"What?" I asked, studying the bright-green silicone mop head.

"I don't know." He shrugged. "The rotisserie?"

I dropped the item in the donate pile since we hadn't used the rotisserie in more than a year, and he'd agreed to get rid of it.

"Hey!" Dean said, snatching it up. "I need that."

"For what?"

He considered it for a moment. "It's cool."

"It goes."

He let his gaze roam over me and then his mouth twisted in a smirk. "I need it."

"For what?" I asked again.

He grabbed a clean tea towel, and lightning fast, he dropped the mop, grabbed my wrists and twisted the towel around them, binding me. I blinked, confused but undeniably turned on.

"For what?" I murmured for lack of something more intelligent to say.

"For this." He walked behind me and pulled my sweatpants down. I was dressed for cleaning—not for sex—but beneath the baggy sweats I was bare.

He pushed me forward, and I rested my wrists on the sink's edge. The brush came down hard on my asscheek, and I yelped. The strands stung more than I'd expected, the silicone tail delivering a stinging bite.

"What's this?" I managed to stutter.

"Punishment for making me get rid of my toys."

My pussy became drenched at the word "punishment."

He lashed me softly with the head of the mop. I found myself flinching at first, but then as the pain faded into a warm, pulsing pleasure, I found myself pushing back, begging for more with my body.

"Look at you," he said, and the words brought a shameful heat to my cheeks.

He stilled the barbeque mop for an instant and slipped a finger into my pussy.

"Soaking wet," he declared, wiggling his finger deep inside me. I bit my lip and tried to focus on not coming undone. I was shocked at my reaction, and yet, I reveled in the sensation. It was freeing.

He pushed a second finger into my cunt and proceeded to fuck me very, very slowly. I realized I was holding my breath, trying to focus on and capture every flicker of stimulation he was delivering.

"Lean forward." I obeyed, but he insisted, "More."

I followed his command instantly, leaning over the sink even farther with my hair hanging down and my ass out.

Dean worked a third finger into me and thrust up hard. He filled my pussy, and my heart skittered.

His other hand worked a steady rhythm with the tool. Slap, slap, slap—pause. Then his fingers tormented me again, thrusting and curling.

I was panting, my fingers warring with themselves inside my bonds as I rocked my body backward, taking everything he was giving and wanting more.

Dean pulled his fingers free and turned me around. "Lean back against the sink, thighs wide."

The stern set of his mouth and the harsh commands all coupled with the impromptu punishment and finger-fucking made me mind-less with lust. I wanted to grab him, undo his belt and beg him to fuck me, but the tea towel prevented me. Instead, I struck the pose he required and waited, chewing my lower lip to keep myself quiet.

He closed the distance between us and kissed me roughly. "You know what I have to do, don't you?"

I shook my head, but I knew. And it filled me with a touch of dread and a great deal of arousal.

"You know—just a few. You'll be fine. In fact, you'll love it."

Dean slapped my pussy with the mop. The small, silicone head kissed my clit with a spark of fire. I moaned.

He did it again. And again. I counted eight total until I was sagging against the lip of the sink. My head was tossed back, my eyes half-closed and my hair a mess.

"Please, Dean," I whispered. "Please just...*something*."

He grinned wickedly and sank to his knees. "I'll make it better," he said. "Because you behaved."

His mouth was soft and giving, and when he lapped at my clitoris, I shuddered. He sucked and soothed, licked and nudged, over and over until sweetness filled me and I hummed softly with mindless joy.

He grabbed my wrists and tugged me down before removing the towel. Dean maneuvered me so that my hips were straddling his head and my face hovered over his crotch. I took his cue and shoved his shorts down and then his boxers. I took his cock in my mouth as his fingers skimmed the tender skin of my ass. He pushed on a particularly hot spot, and I gasped. He shoved a moist finger in my ass as his mouth returned to my slit. His tongue did its thing so beautifully that I arched up mindlessly to intensify the contact.

I sucked down to the root of him, grinding my cunt against his face and loving the strokes of his fingers over my tortured bottom. The digit in my ass drove deeper, and I knew I'd come soon.

I dragged my tongue along the rim of his cockhead before teasing the slit in the top. Precome coated my taste buds, a subtle flavor that always made me smile. I ran my open lips down the sides of his cock and worked his shaft with my hand as he continued to eat me.

He drove his tongue against my wet sex and then licked my pounding clitoris again. He delivered a single slap to my asscheek, inflaming the already sensitive skin, and I came. My body went rigid, the air leaving my lungs. I was frozen in time for an instant as I trembled above him, his big arms hooked around my thighs to hold me steady.

I went back to sucking him off, and he resumed his work on my slit. "No," I mumbled. "Too much."

"Not so," he answered, thrusting up from beneath me and filling my throat. I sucked his cock, tasting the salt-and-cotton flavor of him. I moaned, and the rumble of my voice made him grow still for an instant as he focused on the pleasure.

I put all my efforts into making him come, and when the inevitable conclusion began, he was back at my clit, delivering hard, smooth circles with his tongue.

I inhaled before getting my mouth all the way down his shaft. My lips brushed his pubic hair, and the feel of him filling my throat was sublime. Dean came hard, his cream flooding my mouth. Then he nipped my clitoris and I came again, carried away by the intensity and the surprise of my orgasm.

I rolled off him and picked up the discarded basting mop. I studied it for a moment.

He leaned on his elbow, watching me, and asked, "Well?

Verdict?" The commands and stern face were gone. The dominant man telling me what to do was once again my smiling, joking husband.

"We can keep it."

He laughed. "Excellent. You know it's cool. I just proved it."

My Wife's Playmate

Benjamin Eliot

I was the one to approach Nick. Dana usually chooses the guys, but after getting to know him while hanging out in the local pub, I had become fixated on seeing him with my wife. I told her all about him, and then I asked her if she'd mind me propositioning him.

Not surprisingly, my wife told me to go for it. If it would turn me on, it would turn her on. And then everyone would be happy.

After work one night, I sat with Nick shooting the shit over some local microbrews. Finally, I found that sweet spot in the conversation and brought it up. The idea of watching him fuck Dana.

"You sure about this, man?" he asked. He didn't seem put off, but he did seem wary.

"Trust me, you wouldn't be the first. It's sort of our thing," I replied, keeping the offer simple.

He turned his beer 'round and 'round on the coaster, thinking. Then he said, "What the hell, right? Count me in."

I went home and told Dana immediately. She was all over me and jacked my cock to full hardness before climbing on board. I held her big breasts in my hands, watching her face as she brought herself to orgasm, and then I began to imagine what she'd look like with Nick's cock in her mouth. And that's when I came.

Nick arrived Friday night with a bunch of flowers, of all things. Dana found it very sweet and amusing. So much so, I thought she'd have his pants off before we left the foyer. But she did manage to invite him in and ask him if he wanted a drink. He declined.

"It's my first time doing this, so the sooner we get going, the less chance there will be of me losing my nerve."

"Well, we wouldn't want that, would we?" my wife responded, hiking up her long white skirt and straddling his lap right there on the sofa. She sifted her fingers through his light brown hair. "Now don't panic, but I'm going to kiss you."

And then she did. My cock stirred. Watching her work her magic with other men never failed to turn me on. I sat back in the side chair, content to watch the show. The building excitement and anticipation took my breath away.

She wiggled on his lap, her arms draped around his neck as she kissed him. He made a sound that was all lust, and I smiled. She had that effect on men.

Dana lifted his shirt and let her fingers run along his abs. She rocked from side to side for a moment before purring, "Oh, I think he has something for me, baby."

I said nothing. I simply bent and took a condom from the

table. She pulled Nick's tee over his head, and he grabbed her hair and yanked her forward for an intense kiss. I watched his hips thrust up because he was excited, and the sight turned me on enough to make my fingers shake. I didn't touch myself though. I never did when she was in the middle of it. I'd wait for the end, and then I'd have my time with her.

Nick grunted, finding his comfort zone, and shoved up her skirt. He'd stopped darting glances my way and was totally focused on Dana. He pushed her panties aside and used his thumb to rub her clit. She clutched her skirt to her waist like some kind of surprised maiden and watched him touch her. She gasped, obviously enjoying his attention.

"I think you need to take those pants off now," she said. "I'm so wet. So very wet, and I need you to do something about it."

She climbed off his lap and pushed her skirt down along with her panties. She tugged her flimsy turquoise blouse off, exposing the bare flesh beneath. I watched silently, enjoying the show when he eventually looked at her naked body. The expression of arousal and concentration was instantly shattered by another expression: lust.

She pulled the button fly of his jeans and tugged hard. First one, then all the other buttons below, surrendered. Then he was scooting his jeans and briefs down, grabbing his cock and holding it straight up. She took the condom from me. She bent to put it on him, but not before lowering her pretty lips down over his dick. His eyes slammed shut, and I watched as she sucked him deep before tonguing his balls.

"Now," she demanded, sitting up and looking him in the eye. She rolled the condom on his shaft and moved to straddle him again. This time when she sank down onto his lap, she was lowering herself onto his erection. I watched his cock disappear slowly and sighed. Good. It was so good.

Nick grabbed her hips, his big fingers biting into the meat as he thrust up under her. He was already reading her body's cues perfectly—already knowing she'd want a bit of rough with her tumble.

She hummed, tossing her head back, and pushed her breast to his mouth. He licked her nipple so gently it tortured her, and she let out a little cry. Nick smiled and then gathered her nipple into his mouth and sucked hard. Dana sighed. I held back my own echoing sound. He used his teeth, and she rocked her body as she clutched his broad shoulders. When he moved to the other nipple and repeated the pleasurable teasing, she came.

Nick's dark eyes were hooded with desire as he watched her ride out her pleasure. Then he stood and moved her to the sofa, positioning her on her hands and knees. Dana waggled her ass back and forth, utterly lost in the moment. She glanced at me over her shoulder and smiled before licking her lips. That let me know what was in store for me. What I could expect. Her mouth on my cock—and then my dick burrowing into her sweet pussy just a brief time after someone else's had been there.

I had to sit on my hands to keep from touching myself.

He plunged into her from behind. Nick placed one hand on the small of her back to anchor her as he pounded into her, rough and eager. He said something in a low voice that I couldn't make out but she could. She put her hand beneath herself and began to strum her clit. I watched her force her body back to take him, and then I watched as he licked his middle finger and pushed it right into her asshole.

She shuddered—eyes closing, hair flying—and came. He

grunted again—the caveman sounds were the best part—and held her hips tight with his free hand. Over and over again he thrust, fucking her ass with his finger until he tipped his head back and bellowed as he climaxed.

We gave him a few minutes to recover, and then I thanked him for coming and asked him if he was interested in returning. I barely finished the question before he was nodding agreement. We hustled him out the door, and then I turned to her.

"Come here," she said, bending a finger at me. "I've had my appetizer. Now I'm ready for the meal."

I nodded, moving toward her.

She waved that finger again. "But first, you need to ditch the pants."

"I'm already there," I said, as I unbuttoned them. "One step ahead of you." When I glanced at her hungry expression, I smiled and added: "Now get on your knees."

Meeting the Neighbors

Lily Aikens

"Oh yes! Oh god, oh yes!"

New town. New job. New apartment. New noises from upstairs on the balcony. I was in the middle of moving into the neoclassical studio apartment with the view of the San Francisco Bay when I started to notice sultry sounds emanating from upstairs.

Maybe if I hadn't taken a breather to arrange my plants I would have dismissed the erotic soundtrack as simply part of the city. But I was really drinking in my fresh environment, pausing to pay attention to every little detail. The move had been momentous for me. I was embarking on a brand-new adventure. So I had my ears perked when I heard what was most definitely a sigh of pleasure followed by a moan of bliss and then a whimper of ecstasy. I stared up, but that didn't help me any. "Up" was the bottom of the balcony above me. My ceiling was their floor. Who they were I didn't know. I hadn't met any of my new neighbors. I sat on the lone chaise lounge to listen further.

There was the same type of sigh again. The sound was decidedly, gloriously female. In fact, I deduced after another moment of eavesdropping, *all* the sounds were most definitely female. This meant that either there was one woman up there on the balcony pleasuring herself loudly, or there were two women upstairs pleasuring each other.

When the sounds became words once more, I held my breath. "Don't stop, Sarah. Please don't stop."

Two women. I smiled at my stellar detective skills. One woman was definitely being taken care of by another. I lay back on the lounge and began to touch myself through my charcoal stretch pants, my fingers instantly encountering slippery wetness at my split. I didn't worry that anyone might see me. My balcony was screened in with bamboo walls on either side. I was up high enough that nobody from the street would have been able to see.

"You like that, Janie?" The second voice was deeper, but definitely female. I started to try to picture what the women looked like. The second woman sounded older than the first to me. That's when I heard a third voice.

"*Of course*, she likes that. She loves when you tongue her clit like that, the dirty girl."

"Three!" I said out loud. And then I bit my bottom lip, wondering if the trio had heard my unexpected exclamation. There was sudden silence from above. Then, as if one of the women had gone on her knees to call down through the slats in the balcony railing, a voice said, "Who's that?"

I didn't know what to do. I stared up at the pale-green tendrils of a spider plant that were hanging down toward my balcony, but they didn't offer any advice. This wasn't how I was planning on introducing myself to my new neighbors, but they had clearly heard me and knew I was there. I sucked in a breath of air and said, "My name's Lily. I'm your new neighbor."

"Well, hey new neighbor," came the warm, deep voice. "Why don't you come upstairs? We're in 512."

I'd left my old life behind. An old job, a miserably damp apartment and a love life so stale I could hardly remember what pleasure felt like. Quickly, I hurried into my apartment, ran a comb through my short hair and pinched my cheeks for color. I looked down at my outfit. Damn. I was in a white V-neck shirt and gray sweats. Under normal circumstances I would've preferred to wear something different. But that would have to do. I hadn't unpacked my pretty clothes yet.

I hurried up the steps to apartment 512. The door was wide open. Inside, three attractive women sat on a white semicircular sofa. They were sipping what appeared to be margaritas. They didn't look like people who had recently made love on a balcony. Well, except for the definite sex vibe in the room. I could almost see the lust in the air. Feeling mildly embarrassed, I introduced myself, and the dark-haired woman on the end of the sofa said, "I'm Jo." I recognized her voice as the baritone immediately. She was tough looking but sexy, in jeans and a black vest. On the other edge was a redhead with braids, who turned out to be Sarah. That made the blonde girl in the middle Janie. I was invited to introduce myself, offered a margarita, and after a few sips, I felt more relaxed.

In a short space of time, I explained that I'd moved to California from the Midwest and was looking forward to a whole new life.

So far so good. That is until Jo said, "So, you were listening in?"

I froze—then nodded.

"Did you like what you heard?"

And I melted. "Yes," I said. "You all sounded so sexy."

"If you thought listening was hot, wait until you see what being part of it is like."

I couldn't believe this was happening. I'd never found myself in a situation even remotely as exciting before. I reminded myself that I was going to grab life with both hands now—that had been my plan. Except it wasn't life I grabbed, it was Jo—and she grabbed me back. Her big, muscular arms embraced me, and we kissed. Oh, sweet heaven. Her lips were delightful, and when she started to French me, I closed my eyes and floated from the sensation. That's when Sarah got involved. She started to touch me from behind, and I felt myself relax into her embrace. Sarah cradled my breasts, and she whispered, "You're not wearing a bra."

"No, I haven't had a chance to unpack any yet," I said, when we paused the kiss to breathe.

"Panties?"

I shook my head. Jo said, "It won't take much to get her naked."

With that, they peeled off my clothes and spread me out on the sandy-beige carpet. I was in shock as Janie got between my legs and Jo began to lick my tits. That left Sarah to move around all of us, touching and kissing and petting here and there.

"We meet every Friday evening," Sarah said as Janie lapped at my clit. "We play around inside and on the balcony, and everyone gets off over and over."

I was so close so quickly. Jo pushed Janie aside and began to slip two fingers up my snatch. Sarah now moved to nip at my swollen clit, and I began to whimper. I knew I sounded exactly like Janie had out on the balcony. I'd rarely ever made noise when making love before—but I'd never been in a scene like this either. *Every Friday—*that's what I kept thinking—*every Friday I might be joining in an orgy. Where I could...*

That's when Janie settled herself on my face, and I began to dine on her pussy. She had pale-blonde pubes, even lighter than the hair on her head. Her juices were delicious, and I focused on lapping up every drop. I was so consumed with her pleasure that I forgot my own for a moment. Until I felt something else inside me, something hard and long and...a motor rumbled to life. I was being fucked with a vibrator! I think I lost it then. I cried out, and the vibrations of my voice brought Janie to her own release. She came, copious sex juices coating my lips, and then she moved off me. Jo immediately licked Janie's sweetness from my mouth, and Sarah continued to work the toy inside me.

I came again, on the cusp of the first orgasm, and I felt all the worries I'd brought with me from the Midwest evaporate. As Sarah poised to take her turn astride my mouth, and as Jo began to kiss Janie at my side, I realized that I was going to get along in my new home just fine.

Special Delivery

Davis Carter

Her groceries intrigued me first. I'm a checker at a top-shelf gourmet market, and I started to notice the items on the asphalt-gray conveyer belt before I even looked at the customer. Expensive champagne, fat purple grapes, fancy cheese, a fresh baguette—these were definitely date foods or party foods. In fact, I'd have hastened to say they were "sex" foods.

Curious, I glanced at the woman in front of me, and I saw she was one of my favorite customers. Chelsea was in her mid-forties, I guessed, but she was far more attractive to me than any of the young starlets who come traipsing through my aisle on a regular basis. She had an athletic style, often clad in yoga wear, her thick, black hair pulled back in a bun, nearly no makeup on her striking face. Her body was rocking—I could see everything beneath the spandex she favored—but it was the sexy banter we shared that I looked forward to the most.

This evening, she shot me one of her cock-hardening smiles that made me grateful for the conveyer belt in front of me. She couldn't tell I was getting aroused as I tallied her groceries. When I told her the total, she handed me the cash and then asked if I would be available for a delivery later.

I was confused. Yes, our grocery store delivers, but why would she want me to bring over one bag? Turns out, she didn't. She grabbed the bag herself, slipped me her address and said, "All I want is you."

Excitement flared through me. I handed her the change and felt an electric charge when our fingers touched. She lifted her bag and walked from the store, and I stared through the windows as she settled into her sports car and drove away.

The last few hours of my shift passed in slow motion. When I clocked out, I bought a bouquet of pale-pink roses, and then I hurried to the address she'd given me. The street she lived on was right on the ocean, only a few blocks from the store. As soon as I pulled up, Chelsea opened the door to her bungalow and motioned for me to come in. She'd clearly been waiting for me.

I walked along her front path, breathing in the scent of the salt air and the fragrance of orange blossoms on the breeze. Chelsea was wearing jeans and a champagne-colored halter in a floaty fabric, casual but still a change from her workout attire. Her dark hair was down from the severe bun she usually favored. She looked breathtaking. I stood in her doorway, dumbstruck, and offered her the roses.

She took the flowers and ushered me into her place. After setting down the bouquet, she pulled her halter over her head and let the fabric flutter to the floor. Then she peeled off her jeans and spun to face me. She had nothing on beneath, and my heart hammered and my dick got hard. I couldn't believe this beautiful woman was standing in front of me naked.

On a table behind her, I saw she'd set out the grapes, cheese and wine. There were candles on the mantel, and soft music played from hidden speakers. Before I could say a word, Chelsea was in my arms and her mouth was pressed to mine. I was embarrassed about my erection, and I tried to keep our bodies slightly apart, but the woman knew what she wanted. She set one palm to the front of my jeans, and as soon as she realized I was erect, she gave a happy little laugh that was surprisingly girlish. "This is what I love about men in their twenties," she said, and when she gazed up at me, I saw heat and lust in her eyes.

"What's that?" I murmured.

"Rock. Hard. Cock."

Christ, the way she said the words made me even harder. She seemed so refined that I'd never imagined she would have a dirty mouth. Then she surprised me further by dropping to her knees and opening up my jeans. Talk about a dirty mouth—Chelsea's was open and hungry, and in seconds, I was winning the best blow job I'd ever had.

To date, I'd only been out with women my own age. It had never occurred to me to look to older ladies. Not that I didn't flirt with them, but I hadn't worked up the nerve to make a play. Chelsea obviously didn't mind making the first move in any sense of the word. She was sucking me ravenously from the get-go, and when she paused for air, she said, "You feel so good in my mouth. I can't wait to feel you in my pussy."

I leaked a little precome from the way she was talking. I couldn't get enough of hearing those fuck-me phrases from such a pristine-looking lady. Who would ever have guessed she was so naughty? She seemed like the definition of class. Now, she was standing and leading me to her bedroom. The décor was a blur. I saw art. I saw mood lighting. Then I saw Chelsea's bed.

The huge four-poster took up nearly the whole room. Chelsea practically pounced onto the mattress and then turned to face me. "I want to watch you strip." I got my clothes off faster than I ever had before. When had I last been with a woman as stunning or aggressive? Never. She pulled me to her and soon had me on my back. My dick was pointing straight up, which was perfect, because Chelsea straddled me and sank down all the way to the root of my cock.

We both sighed at the same time.

"I've been waiting for this for so long," she said.

"Me too," I confessed before adding, "I mean, I've been fantasizing about fucking you since I first saw you. But I never thought it would really happen. This isn't a dream, is it?"

She pinched one of my nipples—to prove I was awake—and then raked her nails down my naked chest. That trick made my cock absolutely throb inside her. Chelsea swiveled her hips in a delicious move that had me right on the verge. I didn't want to come yet. I couldn't come yet. I had to prove myself to her—prove my prowess to her. I closed my eyes. I tried to think unsexy thoughts, to no avail. Chelsea said, "Every time I went grocery shopping, I had to drive home as fast as I could to get myself off while thinking of you. I used my favorite vibrator and imagined it was your cock getting me off."

That did it. I came with such force that I almost bounced her off me. Chelsea held on to my shoulders and ground her hips down, maintaining our connection. She didn't seem upset at all by the fact that I'd gotten off. In fact, she slid off my softening dick and spun around so I could lick her pretty split. I'd never done something like that before—eaten out a girl after coming inside her—but Chelsea made me want to do all sorts of unexpected things. As I worked her clit between my teeth, she ever so gently started to suck my cock. I began to harden up again in no time.

But I didn't pay attention to my cock's actions. Right now, I was focused on the honey-drenched treat on my lips. I sucked Chelsea's clit until I felt her body stiffen. I could taste my own come mixed with her juices, and that gave me an extra special charge. Chelsea moaned around my dick, and the vibrations were truly thrilling. I felt her whole body go taut as I suckled her clit. Then she let loose of my manhood long enough to shout, "Oh, fuck, Davis. I'm coming. I'm coming!"

To my delight, the cougar had only gotten started. Still breathing hard, she pulled me around so that I was astride her and she was on her back. Missionary style, I took her once more. She wrapped her long legs around me and held me to her. I felt prouder of my stamina on this coupling. I got Chelsea off two more times before I pulled out and began to simply rub my cock up and down her slippery split. She went out of her head, moaning and purring, arching and growling. When I came for the second time, I made sure we got off together. The experience was transformative. All of my past interactions with women had been sexual intercourse.

This was fucking.

Only after we'd fulfilled our pleasure did we decide to nibble on some of the festive treats Chelsea had set out for us. We needed the fuel for the next round of the night, which took us well into the morning. We made love in ways I had only dreamed about. Chelsea had no problem running me through the paces.

My favorite cougar still shops regularly at the grocery store. Every time she comes through my line, I know I'm going to have a night of sweet satisfaction ahead.

His Bad Girl

Quinn Gabriel

When I need Derrick's hands on me, all I have to do is tell him.

The last time life got too overwhelming, work too insane, I felt that crawling need in my chest, and I picked up my phone.

When he answered, all I had to say was, "I need it, baby."

And that was that.

"Come right home tonight. Forget the grocery store. We'll order in," he said in a deep, husky voice, and then the line went silent as he disconnected.

The hair on the nape of my neck stood on end, and my nipples became stiff little peaks beneath my blouse. I took a deep breath and then was able to carry on with the rest of my day. Sales tickets, vendor phone calls, mix-ups perpetrated accidentally by the new girl—all of those petty concerns bled away because they didn't matter anymore. Very soon, I'd get what I needed.

Derrick was already home when I arrived.

I kicked off my shoes and left my work stuff by the door.

"Come sit on my lap," Derrick said.

He was seated in the large, overstuffed navy-blue chair by the fireplace. The makings of a fire were set up, but the stones were cold, the fire unlit.

I settled myself in his lap and exhaled long and slow as he slid a hand beneath my blouse. His fingers played along the lace of my bra, tickling the skin beneath until I squirmed. Then he pushed the lace down and found my nipple with his fingertips. His lips brushed against mine as he pinched me. When I gasped, he kissed the sound away.

Our tongues played, and when both nipples were bared—the bra cups pushed beneath my breasts—Derrick began to unbutton my blouse. He took his time, making me suffer, building anticipation until it throbbed wetly between my legs like a wicked drumbeat.

Once I was stripped, he dropped my blouse on the floor, bent to kiss the swell of my breasts, and then captured one nipple between his teeth.

He sucked, bit and made me squirm some more. Finally, I captured his head in my hands, angled my body toward him and whispered, "Please, baby."

He grinned, and the vision of him inspired a lust that went straight to the center of me. My cunt flexed from the look on his face. That look said he'd tortured me long enough and now we'd get down to business.

"Okay, then. Get over my lap."

No games. No role-playing. No fucking around with wooing. The act was as simple as breathing. If I wanted a spanking, I asked. And he was more than happy to deliver.

I draped myself across his thighs, feeling my insides grow wetter as he pushed my skirt up around my hips, baring my panties and my ass. I wore plain old boring hose, and he yanked those down, wrestling with them until they were off and in his hand. Then he tossed them toward the fireplace with a chuckle.

"God, I hate those panty hose."

I snorted. "Me too. But I was in a hurry. They were the first ones I grabbed."

"I guess that's why we're spanking you. You've been a bad, bad girl, wearing those ugly stockings." There was a smile in his voice.

He began with my panties up, delivering short, soft swats that barely did anything except rev me up. I moved my hips from side to side, shameless and desperate. I wept openly from nothing but need.

"Derrick," I whispered. "Jesus...please."

His hand came down a bit harder, striking my right cheek firmly enough that an electric jolt seemed to travel beneath my skin, heating my blood. A second blow descended on the same cheek when I expected him to alternate. My breath caught. "Never predictable," he said, dragging his finger up my asscrack, shoving my plain white panties against my skin.

I humped at his lap, bit my lip and prayed for mercy.

He sensed my need because he hooked his fingers into the sides of my panties and pushed them down over my hips. When the undies were midway down my thighs he left them there, a cotton form of bondage.

His fingers found my wetness, and he drove two digits into me from behind. The penetration nearly put me over the top, and I whimpered, caught on the verge of orgasm and emotional release.

"Stay still now," he said. He began to spank me in earnest. Left, right, left, right, the blows taking my breath away until the hot, bright pain transitioned coolly into a heady pleasure.

On the tenth blow, he found my clitoris with his finger and stroked wet circles across the hard knot of flesh until I came, shuddering and sobbing against his legs.

Then he began spanking me again.

He swatted me lightly, tapping with his fingertips against the punished skin that beat in steady time with my heart. I found myself rising up to meet his blows, and when my hips would sink, I'd feel the ridge of his thighs beneath my sex.

We kept up that routine until I turned my face toward him and said, "Fuck me, baby."

And then the spanking became the thing that had already happened instead of the thing I needed to happen. He pulled me onto his lap, so that I was straddling him. I worked open his buckle and zipper, and when he held his cock up for me, I sank down onto his shaft with a ferocity that made us both laugh.

My fingers gripped his shoulders, and he held my hips tight in his hands as I moved up and down, impaling myself with enough force to steal my breath and make my stomach drop like I was falling. I rode him frantically until his jaw clenched and his breath came sharply.

When he reached behind me and delivered a stinging smack to my still-smarting ass, I came with a loud cry that he instantly mimicked with one of his own. Then he pressed his forehead to mine and kissed me.

"Did you get what you wanted, little girl?"

"And then some." I kissed his neck. "Until I need it again."

He gathered my hair in his hand and tugged lightly, just enough to tilt my head back and bare my neck, so he could deliver a soft love bite.

"When that happens, you know where to find me."

Come Here Often?

MARSHA LEWIS

I met Jessica at a party and couldn't take my eyes off her the entire night. I was fresh out of a bad relationship and had just finished divvying up belongings with my girlfriend. The last thing I needed was another woman in my life, but Jessica was beyond gorgeous in a stunning punk way, and I was completely fixated.

My friend Amy told me Jessica wasn't attached. That only made my desire worse. Watching Jessica play with the toothpick full of olives in her martini had my panties wet. The way she kept licking the olives without actually eating any made it impossible not to imagine her mouth on me. Or maybe how those long fingers would feel sliding into my cunt.

"You need to go hit on her already, Marsha," Amy insisted.

"You're looking pretty pathetic standing here salivating over her."

I gave Amy a swat but took her advice. I made my way over and tried some small talk.

"Nice hair," I said, before introducing myself. Her hair was a long mass of purple and pink. I figured it was the worst pickup line in the history of the world.

"Thanks. It takes a lot of work to make hair look this bad."

Her eyes were big and blue and clear like a fall sky. My lust increased.

"I mean it," I said, taking a strand of her long hair and tugging. I watched her eyes grow wide and her lips part in the most decadent way. I couldn't tell if I'd turned her on or if she was going to clock me one.

"Want to get out of here?" she asked.

I opened my mouth and then shut it. Well, that answered my question. Finally, I managed a soft, "Sure."

We walked out into the crisp night. Jessica led me to the back of the property where the owner had built a gazebo. "In here."

My heart skipped a beat, but I followed her. The gazebo was dark and held a few plush lounge chairs. She turned to me and seemed to fly into my arms. Then she kissed me, her mouth soft and sweet and a bit salty from the olives.

"I don't really know you, but I'd like to..." She trailed off and shook her head, like she was talking herself out of speaking.

"Like to?" I felt my heart give another kick, and then her hands were caressing the front of my velvet leggings, and I thought I might go into full-blown cardiac arrest.

"Like to do this," she said, petting my pants again. Another kiss, and I saw colors flash behind my closed eyelids.

Her hand slid down into my pants and found me wet. She kissed me again, and I gently sucked her tongue, wanting to bite but afraid I'd scare her. When she moaned into my mouth, I did it anyway. She pushed herself against me, her fingertip skating over my clit. I thrust my hips forward, liking how she touched me. Wanting more.

She shoved her hand deeper into my pants and slipped three fingers into my slit. My cunt was so wet that her fingers went in with ease. It was my turn to moan now.

She lowered her head and sucked my nipple through my thin white tee. I was braless, and my nipple responded instantly, going hard in her mouth. She nipped it with her teeth, and my cunt flexed around her thrusting fingers.

"Get on a chair," I said, my voice heavy with lust.

Jessica dropped to a chaise lounge, and I tugged off her faded skinny jeans. I pulled her panties down, and when she was bare I dropped to my knees and went right for her pussy. I'd have kissed her thighs, her hip bone, her belly, but she'd gotten me revved up and there was no time for niceties. I wanted to taste her before I lost my mind and my nerve.

I put my mouth on her. She was sweet and salty, and she raised her trim hips up to meet my lips. She wasn't shy in the least. I dragged my tongue along her outer labia, swept it over her swollen clitoris. I nudged that hard knot of flesh repeatedly with my tongue until she was squirming. Then I shoved my fingers inside her and felt the hot, silky grip of her sex.

"That's nice," she said sweetly, and my heart fluttered.

I had forgotten this part. How good sex could be. How good that connection could feel.

I put all my warm feelings into eating her. I sucked her clit and followed with repeated swishes of my tongue. When she was purring like a cat, I nipped her with my teeth again. She jumped, laughed, and motioned with her fingers. "Get up here. Let me have some, too."

I slid my leggings down and straddled her head. When her mouth brushed over me and her breath heated me, I remembered why sixty-nine is my lucky number.

Jessica pushed her tongue into my wet opening and then lavished my clit with kisses and licks. I was on the verge of coming already and tried to focus on using my mouth on her to stave off the orgasm. Somewhere in the party someone laughed loudly. I smiled, sucking Jessica's clit again, driving my fingers inside her deeper. I tried not to grind too far down on her face, not wanting to steal her air, but she grabbed my ass and tugged me closer, burying her face in my pussy, licking me like she'd die if I didn't come.

Her fingers jammed inside me again, and she fucked me with a rough but steady rhythm that took my breath away.

I felt her grow tighter around my fingers, tasted how much sweeter she got closer to orgasm. I concentrated on her clit, nudging it over and over again with my tongue. She mimicked me with her mouth on my pussy. She grew even tighter around my thrusting digits and then said, "Oh yeah. Oh, like that. I'm going to—"

She was coming before she finished the sentence but trying her best to give my clit attention between whimpers. Her sounds died off, and she sucked me in, released me, sucked me in, and released me. My head was reeling, and right when I thought I'd start to beg, she circled my clit over and over again with that amazing little pink tongue and my body surrendered to the pleasure.

I came with a stifled cry, my body shaking violently above hers. She licked me a few more times very softly, and I almost came again.

When I sat up, she grabbed me and kissed me once more, licking her own juices off my lips. A spotlight came on near the house, most likely triggered by partygoers or maybe a curious animal. Jessica smiled in the soft white glow and then laughed.

"What?" I asked, waiting for my heart to calm down a little.

"Would it be cliché if I said: So…do you come here often?"

I laughed. "Would it be cliché if I offered to take you inside and get you a drink?"

She nudged me playfully with her elbow. "I do believe I could be talked into another."

I was hoping she wasn't just referring to the drink. Turned out I was in luck. We had another drink and then revisited the gazebo.

A Playful Getaway

VIVIAN ARIAS

I thought we were going hiking, so when Richard texted me to meet him in the woods at the red bench, I thought nothing of it. The red bench was something we'd stumbled over about halfway up a barely used three-mile-long hidden trail.

I got dressed rather quickly and tied on my best, most comfortable hiking boots. I grabbed a hydration pack, filled it with water and drove out to the state park we hiked most often.

The trail was silent. It was fairly early on a Sunday morning. I walked along quietly, listening to the cicadas in the trees as I headed toward our meeting spot.

I didn't see Richard when I rounded the bend. The bench was empty. Somehow I'd beaten him there. No big deal. I could wait on the bench.

I sat and tilted my head back to catch the trickle of sunlight filtering through the thick canopy of trees. I heard a stick snap and smiled, figuring Richard was there. And he was. I knew when he walked up behind me and rested one big, warm hand on my throat.

"Good morning, pet."

I opened my eyes because "pet" was our keyword for kinky sex and we were exposed on a hiking trail. When my vision came into focus, he dangled several lengths of bright-turquoise nylon rope in front of me. "I think you need to take all those clothes off."

"I...here?" I asked softly. Excitement and dread slithered through me in equal measure.

"Yes. Here."

"But someone might see," I said. My voice had a slight tremor in it.

"True. I think that adds to the deliciousness of the experience. Don't you?"

Easy for him to say. He wasn't going to be the one buck naked and exposed if some other hikers came bouncing down our trail.

"I—"

"You can always say no," he said. Then he walked around the front of the bench to face me. "Go on. Just say no."

I didn't want to say no. I never found myself wanting to say no to Richard. It's why we worked so well together. It's why the sex was off the charts.

I shook my head and saw a flicker of disappointment in his eyes until I stood and pulled my T-shirt over my head. After removing my boots and socks, I shucked my cargo pants and my plain white panties. Bare-ass naked, I sat back down when he indicated I should do so.

"Spread your legs and put your arms behind the back of the bench," he said.

I obeyed him as an early summer breeze brushed across my exposed pussy. My clitoris thrummed with the pleasure of being so wonderfully exposed. So deliciously bare.

He moved behind me, and I felt the intricate coiling of rope upon my skin. Knots and loops and whorls. I couldn't see what Richard was doing, but I imagined the pattern to be exactly what it always is when Richard binds me. Art.

I shut my eyes and tried to calm my racing heart. If someone came, Richard could wave them off. Or toss his button-down over me. Or I could burst into flames from embarrassment. The last thought sent energized terror jolting through my stomach.

I wriggled.

"Stay still," he said. "You need to trust me."

I did trust him. He knew I did. His words had been a simple reminder to calm me.

When he was done, he stepped to the front again and studied me. "Gorgeous."

I wriggled again.

He cocked his head as if he'd heard something, and my heart seemed to stutter in my chest. Then he shook his head. "Musta been an animal. But let's see what that did, shall we?"

He moved toward me, dropping to his knees and pushing his fingers against my pussy lips. He spread me wide and dragged his fingertip along my soaking-wet slit. Then he took the gathered moisture and spread it around my swollen clit. I bucked before I realized I was going to move. My body jerked up to meet the pleasure he delivered, and he smiled.

"Do you have any clue how gorgeous you are?" Before I could answer, he leaned in and licked my left nipple. Then he sucked until it went rigid in his mouth. His teeth took over from there, and he bit me hard enough to trigger a rush of wetness between my legs. Then he tugged my nipple out as far as he could and slid a finger inside me.

I moaned.

Off in the woods something moved, and I felt fresh fear crash down on me. But when Richard shoved a second finger in my pussy, I felt how the possible danger of discovery had aroused me.

He smirked at me. "Do I have a secret exhibitionist on my hands?" He curled his finger, and I sobbed plaintively. "Or not so secret, maybe?" Richard continued.

He put his mouth on my pussy and sucked my clit only long enough to bring me to the razor-sharp edge of orgasm. Then he stopped.

He pushed a third finger in me. I was so wet, my body readily accepted the extra digits. Then he fucked me with his fingers while watching my face for signs of orgasm. When his thumb rested on my clit, and he began to press and manipulate it, I lost control. The orgasm slammed me, ripping a cry from my throat before I even realized I'd reached my limit. Pleasant warmth and heaviness invaded my limbs, and I gasped. "I'm sorry! I'm sorry!"

He tsked at me. Standing and unzipping his fly, he pushed his cock against my lips and I lapped at it greedily. My shoulders screamed from how he had me bound, but I welcomed the discomfort to sharpen my focus. My pussy continued to spasm, aftershocks of my orgasm shattering me.

I sucked him deep, and he held my head in his big hands as he precariously perched on the bench, his knees between my widespread thighs. He fucked my mouth so hard the motion stole my breath. His face grew serious and he drove deeper, filling my throat. I inhaled air into my lungs through my nose and sucked and licked as hard as I could. I wanted to make him come. Drink him down. Please him.

The rope bit into my skin, and I felt a fresh rush of fluid in my cunt from the pain.

"Swallow," he said, and then he climaxed.

I swallowed as fast and as much as I could, and some of his come still slipped down my chin. He wiped off the cream with his thumb.

I heard a voice and was instantly panicky.

"Relax," he said. "They're far off. Let's see if you can come again before they get here."

Richard knew what he was talking about. The other hikers were probably ten minutes away. I was horrified and yet turned on. He dropped to his knees and pushed his hot mouth against my wet pussy. His tongue invaded me, sweeping along my outer lips, targeting my clit until I found myself biting my bottom lip hard enough to hurt.

He sucked that tender bit of flesh over and over, and just when I thought we'd be found, he delivered a hard lick with his flattened tongue, and I came. I cried out, forgetting myself, scaring the small animals in the brush.

Richard laughed and stood. He put himself together, taking his time as he zipped up and straightened his clothes. Then he began to unwind me as I practically vibrated on the bench. The voices were getting closer.

When I was undone, he gave me my pants and I hurriedly got

dressed. I was still zipping up when a group of people rounded the corner.

"Morning!" a woman called. "Beautiful weather isn't it?"

Richard winked at me, giving me a knowing smile. "We think so!" he called, and then he waved to her as we took our leave.

Boss Lady

KITTY WINSTON

Bennie was late for work again. When it's only you and one other person running a very small travel agency, that sort of behavior tends to get old. I took in the circles beneath his eyes combined with the fact that he was a little pale. He was yawning constantly, and I only had one conclusion: late night. Bennie had been out partying, and I was the one now paying the price. My agency, my rules, my loss if he wasn't up to par.

We had about two hours before our next scheduled appointment. When he took his seat with a mumbled, "Morning," I got up and flipped the OPEN sign to CLOSED, then lowered the venetian blind.

"What's up?" I asked.

Bennie is a handsome man. We'd fucked more than once.

Boring summer days with no foot traffic can make for creative ways to pass the time. We both knew getting involved was a bad idea, but fucking was not the same as being involved. Fucking was recreation. And in the travel business our bread and butter was all about recreation.

"Late night. Sorry. Won't happen again." He turned his computer on and waited for the machine to come to life.

"You said that last week," I reminded him. "And the week before."

He sighed and ran a weary hand over his face. His light-brown hair stood up in corkscrews when he shoved his fingers through it. The move was endearing, but I pressed my lips together so he wouldn't be able to see that I thought so.

"I'm sorry. Truly. I'm just..." He shrugged. "I guess I'm restless lately. So I go out with my friends. They all work for themselves so they stay out to ungodly hours, and I try to keep up. I really am sorry. I promise, cross my heart, that it won't happen again," he said, making an *X* on his chest with his finger.

I smiled. "Fine. I'd like you to go grab me the box of brochures for the Caribbean. We need to restock the pamphlets in the front."

He rose, giving me an agreeable nod. Until I said, "And I'd like you to do it on your knees."

His eyes went from dull to sparkly, and the pulse at the base of his throat twitched. I saw him stand up a little bit straighter. But he didn't move.

"You heard me," I said. Then I swatted him on the ass to get him moving. "Do it."

I could tell by the way he adjusted himself that he was hard. He dropped to his knees and crawled back toward the storage room. I watched him go—nice taut ass in a pair of dark-wash jeans. I smiled. The day was looking up.

By the time he'd returned, shuffling across the floor on his knees while holding the small box of pamphlets, I'd located his ruler, a bright yellow strip of wood adorned with black numbers and the contact info for a local plumber.

"Before you fill that up, I believe you owe me a bit of ass for being late. Again," I said sullenly, tapping my knee with the ruler. I kept my face stoic because I didn't want him to know how much fun I was having. Or how turned on I was.

His face fell, but his eyes gleamed. He was torn. Should he fear the pain or anticipate the pleasure? It was my favorite part of playing with Bennie. He was such an emotional guy.

"Come on," I said, pointing with the ruler. "You heard me. Get over here."

He obeyed, shuffling over fast enough that I didn't have to reprimand him. When he was at my feet, I touched his stubbly cheek and said, "Sorry, sweetie, sometimes we all need to learn a lesson."

I positioned his body so he was bent over the seat of his swivel chair, and then I told him to undo his pants. When he had, I tugged the jeans down so his ass was exposed. My initial urge was to bite him on the butt, but I stifled that. If I bit him, we'd be fucking on the floor in moments. Before the fucking he had to pay the piper.

With his bottom bare, I thought for a moment. "Twenty minutes late. I think that's one stripe per minute. Seems fair, yes?"

I tapped the back of his thigh to make sure I had his attention. He didn't answer, and I tapped him again. "I asked you a question."

He nodded fast, pushing his ass back as if asking for it. I saw him thrust once against the empty space beneath the seat. No relief there. I smiled.

"Yes," Bennie said. "Yes, Ma'am."

"There you go," I said, and then I brought the ruler down fast and hard four times in a row.

Bennie let out a cry and did that humping thing again. My pussy was aching from his display. I had to bite the tip of my tongue to keep myself in punishing mode.

"Say something," I commanded.

"I'm sorry."

"Good. You should be." I let the ruler fall four more times, crisscrossing the red area I'd already striped.

He moaned, and I found myself dripping wet. As punishment for his turning me on so badly, I delivered four sharp blows. *That's twelve*, I thought. *Eight to go.*

My pussy was throbbing, slick and desperate. Ready for the orgasm I was going to demand from my employee once we were done.

"Something else," I said.

"It will never happen again."

"It had better not," I said, bringing the ruler down once for every word. I reached beneath him and gave his cock a single stroke, just to torture him. *Four strokes left.*

"I promise," he said, voice explosive in the silent office. Only the hum of the fan on his computer warred with his voice.

Four more fast blows. I watched the redness blossom like a flower on the fair skin of his ass. I could almost, if I concentrated, count the strokes there on his flesh.

I spread my legs and tugged my panties to the side beneath my black skirt. "Come here and make it up to me," I demanded. He moved fast then, his big body in motion as he almost blindly came toward me. He buried his face at the apex of my thighs, lavishing my pussy lips and clitoris with kisses and licks. I arched up, yanking his hair in my hands as I drove myself against his mouth.

"I promise," he said again, his voice muffled by my sex.

"Shut up," I said not unkindly. And then I pushed my pussy up to meet his mouth. His tongue was a flurry of wet motion, and when he sucked my clit hard, I saw stars. He did it again and then again, and finally I was powerless to stop myself. I came with a big sigh, and my body twitched from the pleasure.

When he sat back, sex-drunk and smiling, I nodded toward his cock. "Go ahead," I said. "Get off. It will wake you up some. We have a lot to get done today, and I expect nothing less than 110 percent from you. We'll fuck later."

He jacked his cock hard and fast. Just four rough strokes did the job. He came with a barrage of curse words, his thick white come running down over his fist. "Yes, Ma'am," he said, shaking a little from his release.

"Damn straight—yes, Ma'am," I said, thinking we had a long boring day ahead of us and I might want to revisit his punishment before six o'clock. I patted his head and smiled. "Good boy."

A Real Handy Man

Max Smith

I liked to watch Carson with Savannah. He worked for my independent appliance-repair service, and when my girl was around, poor Carson got rather tongue-tied. He's older, silver haired, big. Handsome in a rugged, outdoorsman kind of way. Of course, Savannah was oblivious to his interest. She'd just swish her long dark hair around, flash her soulful brown eyes and smile at him. Oblivious.

That's until one night, mid-fuck, I broached the subject with her.

"Carson?" she asked. "*Our* Carson?"

"Yep. Our Carson. And I've been thinking. A lot. About him with us."

She just looked at me. "What? Like a threeway?"

"Like a threeway."

"But that would mean me and him and me and you and you know...you and him."

I nodded. "Carson has made the occasional comment that makes me think he'd be down with that."

I sucked her nipple into my mouth and drew on it hard. She squirmed beneath me, and I feared I'd come right there. She arched up beneath me, her pussy clenching tight around my cock. "I'd like that. To see him sucking your cock or something," she murmured. "And if you're interested in seeing me with him, then I could be persuaded."

Her voice was a purr, her cunt slick and hot around me. She squeezed me with her internal muscles, and I went about persuading her.

When I brought the subject up with Carson a few days later, he simply stared at me. A bit of sandwich still filled his mouth, and I had a brief moment where I heard Savannah in my head. *I'd like to see that. To see him sucking your cock...*

I wasn't sure if it was the idea of a man doing that to me or the thought of her enjoying the show, but I found myself aroused.

"Won't it weird things up between us all?" he finally asked, scratching his silver hair. Small lines around his eyes served to give him the appearance of great kindness.

"I don't think so. But if that's a fear of yours, I understand. Just say no."

He blinked, wiped his mouth and shrugged. "Why say no when you can say yes? I'm sure my admiration for your woman hasn't gone unnoticed."

I laughed. "Why do you think I asked you?"

We set it up for Saturday afternoon. He'd come over, and we'd all see where our chemistry led us.

The day finally arrived, and Savannah came downstairs in white shorts and a white tank. It was clear from a glance that she had nothing on underneath, which I found utterly hot. I loved her body, loved her fierce independence and her wicked sense of humor. I equally loved the idea of her displaying all of that to another man, knowing all the while that she was mine.

I ran my hands up and down her ass, her sides, her back. I kissed her. "I like the look. A lot."

I cupped her mound through her shorts and drove my finger along the cleft of her pussy. She swatted me. "Don't touch the goods until the guest arrives!" But I felt her move against my seeking finger. I felt her breath stutter in her chest.

Just then the doorbell rang. I let Savannah answer. I watched Carson take her in and saw the color flood his cheeks.

Once he was inside, I offered him a drink, but he refused. He put his hands nervously in his pockets. Savannah smiled and shook her head. "You're so shy," she said, and then put her hand on the waistband of his jeans and stood on tiptoe to kiss him.

He had to stoop to kiss her, given he was over six foot four. Her hand moved restlessly over his zipper.

"Now, the rumor is my husband would like to see me with you. And have you with us. Game?" Even as she waited for his answer, she was unzipping him.

Carson's eyes drifted shut, and he nodded. It was his only response, but it was enough.

I watched my wife pull his cock free and get down on her

knees, with Carson following suit soon after. She took his dick in her mouth within a heartbeat and began to suck. Carson moaned and put his hands on her head. I watched her ass wiggling the way it did when she was turned on. And she was turned on, I was sure. Because I sure as hell was.

I moved in behind her, reached between her legs and found the crotch of her shorts soaked with her own juices. I did my best to take them off without disturbing her, and then I got down on my knees behind her and slipped my fingers into her pussy.

Up close, it was even better. I could see her glossed lips sliding up and down his shaft. I could hear her breathing and smell her perfume. Carson rocked into her mouth, eyes still shut. When he opened them to find me so close, he looked momentarily stunned, but I smiled and nodded, and he began to more aggressively thrust. I slid my cock into her drenched cunt and began to fuck her. She was tight and wet and excited because every minute or so she would clench up around me to give me an added jolt of friction.

"Don't you come," I told him. He nodded in a half-assed response.

"You," I said to Savannah, reaching beneath her to stroke her distended clitoris. "*You* come."

I fucked her hard, and every thrust drove her generous mouth forward on his dick. She was damn near deep-throating him when she climaxed. Her cunt flexed, milking my cock. He gasped, and I said again, "Don't!"

He nodded quickly and pulled his cock from her mouth. "Then I have to…pause."

"That's good. That's fine." I stood, pulled a condom from my pocket and tossed it to him. My own cock throbbed, so close to orgasm but denied the final climax.

I took a breath and said, "Put that on. Then you get over here and fuck her. You're going to finish up, and then you're going to finish me up." I touched his hair, and Savannah moaned. The sound sent a quick thrill up my spine.

She got on her back, thighs spread wide, and he climbed on top of her. When he thrust into her, she squealed, and he cursed softly, "Christ."

Savannah wrapped her long legs around him, and I moved forward on my knees, my cock nearing his lips. He leaned forward and took my dick into his mouth, and the act turned me on more than I'd imagined it would. I bucked roughly as he sucked and gagged. He kept at it, though, and his thrusts into my wife's pussy grew more intense and demanding.

She arched up under him, crying out as an orgasm hit her. I had to grit my teeth to hold on then, but I did. As his rhythm grew faster and faster, I fucked his mouth harder. The slide of his tongue, the scrape of his teeth, all kept me on the edge of coming.

Carson slammed into Savannah, and she hooked her ankles behind his back. She played with her breasts and hummed softly as he grew closer to climax. When he sucked hard and grunted, groaning around my dick, I knew he was coming. His body grew rigid, but I held his head with both hands and drove into his throat. Savannah gave another cry, a bonus orgasm no doubt, and I let myself go, emptying into his willing mouth as his teeth grazed my shaft.

When we disentangled, Carson sat back, stunned and disheveled. Savannah crawled onto my lap and kissed me. I massaged her breast and pinched her nipple.

"Can you stay for a bit, Carson?" she asked softly. "I have a few more things I'd like to try."

Carson nodded. "Sure. I can do that. No problem."

She looked at me and smiled. All I could do was smile back at her. Our first foray into kinky sex had been a huge success.

Girl Crush

Maria Stewart

Sheila was the girl I hung out with when I visited family in Connecticut. She was tall and fair and liked to wear her hair in two long braids. She was the same age as me, and her hair was the color of lemon cream. I crushed on her for ages until I turned twenty-one. That was the year my crush became my lover.

We were out on the lake with a bunch of other people, but Sheila and I had gone out to the float alone. Her swimming in crisp even strokes, me doing the breaststroke because it was the only way I could swim with any speed. She was like some mythical mermaid. I felt like the beast that attacks the submarine in the horror movies.

We pushed up onto the worn wood and immediately sprawled on our backs. I flung an arm over my eyes to blot out the intrusive, blinding sun. We lay there for a few minutes feeling the bob and dip of the water, and then she took my hand.

"I was glad you came back this summer. I didn't think you would."

I tried to find my voice. It was buried somewhere deep inside me, being held prisoner by my pounding heart and the flushed arousal that had flooded my pussy the moment she touched me.

"Why would you think that?" I managed in response.

She squeezed my hand and then let go. My hand unfurled, flattened palm up to the sun as if exhausted from coming into contact with such an amazing creature. One I'd gotten off to on plenty of nights in my dorm-room bed, making sure to be quiet so my roommate wouldn't hear.

When her finger began drawing spirals on my palm, I was glad my arm was over my eyes so I wouldn't have to look. I could lie there and bite my lip and feel her touch sink deep into my flesh until I feared I'd come just from her drawing invisible marks on my skin.

"We grew up. We're getting jobs," she said matter-of-factly. I finally peeked at her through one squinted eye, and she shrugged. "I figured it would all come to its eventual end, is all."

"Well…I'm here," I finished weakly. "I came."

I pushed my lips together, feeling stupid for my choice of words. But truth be told, if she kept stroking my skin that way, it wasn't a far reach of my imagination to think that I could.

She moved so suddenly I didn't have time to think or to brace myself, which was good. It was as sincere as moments get in a lifetime.

She kissed me. Her face pressed close to mine, her lips cool from the water. She kissed me, and when the kiss grew more intense,

I parted my lips to let her small, soft tongue slide against mine. She pushed her fingers to my belly, and my lust-warmed skin felt hot in response to her lake-chilled flesh.

Sheila broke the kiss. "All those jokers will see, and we'll never hear the end of it. Meet me out by the jogging path tonight. By the cave."

I nodded, unable to speak. And then we simply sprawled there in the sun for hours, thighs touching. I don't know what was going on in her head, but my mind was racing. I could barely fathom making it until nightfall.

When I met her later, she was dressed in a dark sweatshirt and cutoff shorts. She smelled like strawberries and coconut suntan lotion. She took my hand and led me back to the cave. It was really just a small grouping of large rocks that formed a deep semicircle, but we'd all nicknamed it "the cave" years ago.

"I brought a blanket."

Before we were even really sitting, we were kissing. And the kiss took on a life of its own. I pushed my hands beneath her sweatshirt, covering her small breasts with my palms. A rush of pleasure coursed through me when I felt her nipples go hard beneath my touch.

Her lips slid down my neck and then she was pushing me back, shoving my T-shirt up and hooking her fingers in my shorts to tug them down. Her lips skittered along my belly, my hip and then lower. When her mouth touched me—the searing, wet heat of it—my entire body arched up to meet her. Her tongue slid along my nether lips, nudged my clit, and when she sucked it into her mouth and scraped that hard knot of flesh with her teeth, I had to stuff my hand in my mouth to keep from crying out.

Sheila pushed my thighs wide, and her fingers circled my wet slit as she licked me. I gripped the blanket tight, trying so hard to keep quiet and not come. She suckled me again, the pressure on my clit nearly overwhelming. She pushed a finger inside me, and when I moaned and moved against her, she added a second.

I listened to her breathing, to the sounds of her mouth on me, as we lay there tangled in the dark. She thrust a third finger deep inside me, and I clenched my internal muscles to add to the thrill. I came when she nipped my clitoris with her teeth, all the sound freezing in my lungs. But my body language told the tale, and she laughed softly, sitting back.

"Take your pants off," I said.

She laughed again. "I know you've never been with a girl. You've never even—"

"Sheila," I sighed. "Shut up and do it."

"Oh, and she's bossy," she said, but I heard the tremor in her voice. The excitement.

Her zipper sounded unbelievably loud. The full moon gave me just enough stark white light to see the sharp contours of her face.

When she was bare from the waist down, I ran my fingers up her thighs. I traced the prominent angle of her hip bones and the lush flare of her hips. The dip of her waist and the small swell of her belly. I parted her nether lips and inhaled the scent of her before lowering my head to taste her. She was sweet and musky, the hard bump of her clit beneath my tongue exhilarating.

I sucked softly, and she groaned a bit harder. When her hips thrust up and she shoved her hands roughly in my hair, I licked her more aggressively. I slid the tip of my tongue along her nether lips, parting her and tasting salt on my tongue.

Then I pushed her legs flat to the blanket, pinning her there, and licked her over and over and over, relentlessly, until she came, whispering, "Jesus, fuck. Fucking hell."

She'd gone from wet to wetter, and I slid my fingers through the lake of wetness. I worked a thick bundle of fingers into her cunt and fucked her, my lips moving softly over her belly and down her slender thighs. She squirmed and bumped against me saying, "Stop, Jesus, stop. You're killing me."

But she didn't mean it, and we both knew it. So I fucked her harder, deeper, rougher with my fingers, and when she went utterly silent, I delivered one final lick across her still-swollen clit and she climaxed again.

She tugged on my hair to urge me upward until we were belly-to-belly, pussy-to-pussy, face-to-face. She kissed me. Her mouth tasted like me, mine like her.

That night is a memory that's seared in my brain. A wonderful, steamy first. I'm heading back to Connecticut to visit my family this holiday season, and I hear Sheila still lives in town. I'm thinking of looking her up. Maybe we can take a walk out by the cave.

Hungry for Pleasure

LAURIE HALL

I met Dana and Greg at a birthday party. They were the power couple. She was gorgeous and tall; he was just as gorgeous and a bit taller. As the party wound down for the night, I couldn't tear my eyes away from them. They were the hosts; we'd all gathered for Brian's birthday. I worked with Brian, and apparently, he was related to Greg.

As the night wore on and I was about to take my leave, I went over to thank the couple for their hospitality. Dana caught my wrist in her elegant hand. She leaned in and whispered, "Before you leave, I wanted to ask you a question."

I was a little confused but perfectly willing to follow her into the study and listen to what she had to say. Although deep down, I already knew. Once she was done speaking, I leaned against the desk. "So why me?"

All that she had said—the invitation she'd just delivered—and that was my question!

She smiled, blue eyes flashing. Then she reached out to touch my wrist, this time with great deliberation, and my mouth went dry. "Because we've been watching you all night."

"You have?"

"We have."

I shook my head, marveling. Of all the beautiful creatures I'd seen that night, I could not understand their attraction to me. But then Greg walked in, six foot three, dark hair and green eyes, and I shook off my negative thoughts. They'd made their decision, and I'd go with it. Because I wanted them, and if they wanted me, who was I to argue?

"When?"

"Tomorrow night? Come for dinner," Dana said. Her cool fingers stroked my arm before she pulled me closer. Then she leaned in, her dark hair falling over her shoulder, and kissed me.

I was supremely aware of the proximity of her husband as her tongue touched mine. When all of my tension drained, I relaxed and she kissed me deeply. Her fingers played at the waistband of my pants. A single finger dipped beneath before she pulled back.

"For dinner," Greg said.

"You'll be the main course."

When I left the party, I felt like I was floating, and my mind never let go of the vivid fantasies of what might happen the following night.

I changed my clothes four times before I went to their place, and almost turned the car around twice to change again. In the end, I decided they were less concerned with what I had on and more concerned with me once the clothes were gone. I pulled into their driveway and noticed the front door was open. When I got out of the car, music could be heard.

I rang the bell and saw Dana peek around the corner and wave me inside. I inhaled the scent of food. Good food.

"There she is," Greg said, coming into the room with two wine-glasses. He handed me one and then clinked his glass against mine. Dana was right on his heels with her own glass in hand.

"We assumed wine was okay," she said.

"It is. It's welcome, in fact." I swallowed three wonderful sips, and then set the glass down. "Not to be an insane person, but can we... can we do this? Before I burst into flames."

They chuckled simultaneously, a trait I'd spotted in a lot of close couples. It made me feel more secure with them; they seemed two halves of a single whole.

"Come on," Dana said. She took my hand and led me toward the stairs. "Greg will lock up the front and meet us upstairs."

When we reached their bedroom—dark walls, a big bed, very few knickknacks—my eyes darted around the room, but hers didn't. Hers were focused on me as she began to unbutton my dress. "I like your breasts," she said. My lips seemed stuck together. I simply watched her hands on me. "It's why I chose you. I'm big. You're little. I like the fact that I can hold your tits in my hands, and nothing is wasted."

She smiled again, and on a whim I rose and kissed her on the mouth. She sighed against my lips and covered my breasts with her hands. I'd gone without undergarments because I was so damn nervous, and for that, I was incredibly grateful to my own anxiety.

Dana had just slid her hand down my side and stroked my hip

when Greg entered. They seemed to work well as a team because Greg peeled off the dress she'd already unbuttoned. I stood there, my dress puddled around my ankles, as he kissed the back of my neck and she slipped a finger inside me. After a few thrusts and subtle curls of her fingers, I was coming, which surprised me. Then they were getting undressed, and though utterly sober, I felt a little drunk.

"Now then, if you don't want to follow where we lead, just speak up."

She directed me onto the bed where Greg lay, naked but for a condom. He leaned forward, and after she helped me straddle his face, he licked my pussy eagerly. His tongue was soft and warm, and within a minute of him eating me and stroking his cock at the same time, I came. The couple seemed magical in regard to orgasms. Either that or this scenario—one I'd never experienced before—was such a turn-on I had a hair trigger.

We shifted positions, and I eagerly settled onto my hands and knees at Greg's behest. A moan slipped out of me when he settled behind me, and then we both hissed when he entered me. Dana climbed onto the bed, spread her legs and pushed her pussy toward me. I didn't think twice; I buried my face between her thighs and parted her nether lips with my tongue. Then I nibbled and licked at her swollen clit, making her grab hold of my hair.

The bite of pain only served to amp up my pleasure. I'd never gone down on a woman before, and I found her supremely sexy and the taste of her intoxicating.

Dana thrust her hips, grinding her pussy against my mouth. I lapped at her, and then sucked, and then continued to alternate, trying to do to her the things that turned me on.

Greg gripped my hips tightly and slammed into me. His thumb penetrated my asshole. I was overwhelmed with my new lovers in the best possible way, Dana, on my tongue, him in my cunt, his finger in my ass. Pushed, pulled and sucked down into a vortex of pleasure. When Greg reached beneath me and stroked my clit with his free hand, I climaxed once more. As I gasped against her pussy, Dana pulled my hair. Her juices spilled over my lips and tongue as she joined me in erotic bliss. Her orgasm seemed to trigger his because he went rigid against me as he cried out with his own release.

I was boneless, exhausted and spent as they held me there in limbo for a moment. Then Dana backed up and kissed me. "Okay?" she asked.

I nodded.

"Can we feed you now?" she asked. Greg withdrew from me but not before smoothing a hand down my back and across my ass.

"Yes."

"Good," Greg chimed in. "We're hoping you'll stay for...a while."

Dana caught my eye. "He means for the night. But first—food."

"First, food," I agreed. But I already knew I'd stay.

Carnal Cravings

Marlie Palmer

I love to suck Jason's dick. Love it. I'll randomly get in the mood to do it, usually when he's not even close to being in the same room as me. I was at work filing papers the last time the urge hit me. I shut my eyes and thought of taking him in my hand, stroking him to hardness, getting on my knees…

I pulled my phone out of my skirt pocket and texted him.

I want to suck your cock.

My phone lit up in moments, and the answer made me laugh.

You won't hear me arguing.

I went in the corner behind the largest filing cabinet. There was just enough room between the end of the cabinet and the wall for a person to stand without being seen. I hiked up my skirt, pushed my hand into my panties and stroked myself to a shuddering, breathless orgasm from thinking about blowing him.

I'll be home at five, I answered, and then straightened my skirt, fluffed my hair and went back to filing. I kept myself occupied with thoughts of sliding my parted lips down the silken length of his shaft. I barely ate at lunch, and my friend Carrie asked me what was wrong. "You're all flushed. Are you sick?"

"Nope. Just preoccupied," I said.

I was surprised I didn't get a speeding ticket while driving home. I was pushing my little Triumph to sixty in a forty zone and kept correcting myself, only to find the pedal to the metal once more. When I pulled into the driveway and saw Jason's truck, I felt my stomach bottom out as if I was falling.

I left my messenger bag behind and only grabbed my purse. I hurried up the walk, my heels clicking in time with my racing heart. The door was unlocked, and I pushed it open with trembling fingers. He was sitting in the big overstuffed chair, wearing a pair of old jeans and a smile. He sipped from a beer and cocked an eyebrow at me.

"Want a drink?"

"Nope." I dropped my bag.

"Hungry?"

"Nope."

He settled the beer bottle on his flat stomach and considered me. "What do you want?"

"You know what I want," I said, my voice a little raspy. You'd think that it was the first time we'd done this, despite being together for more than five years.

"Well, you know where to get it."

I didn't think about it. I dropped to my knees and crawled toward him across the hardwood floor. My nylons whispered as I moved. He hadn't been expecting that, because Jason sat up and watched me approach. He put the beer bottle down on the table and stared at me as I made my way toward him.

"Take the jacket off," he said.

I pulled off my navy-blue blazer and dropped it on the arm of the sofa.

"And the shirt."

I pulled the plain white shell over my head and didn't bother to fix my short blonde hair.

"Leave the bra on," he said. I started to move. "But pull the cups down."

I sat back on my haunches and did as he requested. My nipples stood out in rosy little peaks.

I didn't ask him to unbutton or unzip his pants because I wanted to do it. I wanted to watch his face as I took care of everything.

I pressed my breasts to his knees as I popped the silver disc of his button. I pulled the zipper down slowly, making us both wait. I waggled my ass back and forth, partly to turn him on but also to draw out the suspense. I clenched my internal muscles, feeling small blips of pleasure deep inside me.

"Up," I said softly. He raised his hips, and I tugged his jeans down. Beneath the denim he was bare.

I took him in hand, stroking him slowly and licking my lips. I watched his face. How his eyes got heavy-lidded and his lips pressed together. When he was beyond hard and the tip of his cock was slick with precome, I leaned forward and slid my tongue along the slit in his dick.

He sighed heavily and put a hand on top of my head. The pressure turned me on as much as the musky, salty taste of him.

I dragged my tongue up the underside of his cock, feeling the thick vein there. I pressed my lips to his shaft, teasing him with open-mouthed kisses while my fingertips stroked his balls.

I blew out softly so he'd feel the heat of my exhalations.

He thrust up, his cock gliding along my lips. His action let me know he was tired of being teased. The hand on my head grew heavier, and I happily sucked the cap of his cock into my mouth. I swirled my tongue along the silken skin, listened to the rumble deep in his chest when he groaned. He thrust again and most of his length disappeared into my mouth. I sucked gently but firmly before pulling back to wet the rest of his shaft.

I licked up the side and then down the other, tasting every part of him before lowering my mouth to let him fill my throat.

"Fuck," he said, and I couldn't help but feel pleased.

I sucked and licked and stroked him with my hand, my fist wet from my own spit.

Finally, I got up high on my knees and held his hips with my hands. I pressed down to pin him and slowly took him as deep into my throat as I could. I bobbed on his length; my rhythm grew faster and his fingers threaded into my hair.

"The things I want to do to you…"

I pulled my mouth from his dick and whispered, "Tell me. Tell me."

Then I took him as deep as I could again, my hands pushing down against him. I pulled off, and then lowered my mouth to his balls, licking the soft skin and sucking each one gently into my mouth. Then I went back to deep-throating him, making sure to alternate my actions to keep him on edge.

"I want to fuck you. That's a given—but not until I've gone down on you. Sweetheart, I'm going to eat that pussy until you weep."

I was getting wetter, and I couldn't seem to keep my ass still. I moved it slowly from side to side as he talked.

"I plan to make you beg me to fuck you."

His hand came down on my head to hold me on his cock. I was done alternating, it seemed. He bucked up, filling my mouth and my throat, making my eyes tear a bit.

"And you *will* beg me."

He thrust harder still, and I felt my nipples grow tight against his thighs from excitement.

"After I ram your pussy, I'm going to flip you over, eat your ass, and fuck you there until you scream."

I shivered, and he thrust deeply once more. Then he was cursing, saying my name and driving up from beneath me. His come—hot and salty—coated my tongue, and I pulled back enough to lick him, even as another spurt erupted.

He held my head the entire time, and I relished the feel of his strong hands on me.

I looked up at him, licking my lips. "Did you mean it?" I said, referring to all the things he'd talked about.

He wiped the sticky wetness from my lower lip and smiled. "The countdown has already begun."

I put my head in his lap and smiled.

Welcome to the Neighborhood

CATHERINE MURPHY

Ed moved into our neighborhood just as fire-pit season was upon us. We invited him over, as good neighbors should, and plied him with hard cider and homemade cinnamon cookies. Dan, my husband, didn't take long to wink at me. He'd seen me studying our new handsome neighbor and obviously approved of my interest.

Ed's very tall and very broad. He has big blue eyes and dark hair, and when he smiles, his lip curls and it sort of reminds me of Elvis—which had a lot to do with how rampantly my lust consumed me after meeting him.

That first night after Ed went home, Dan pulled out a big stinky cigar and waggled his eyebrows at me as he puffed the cherry on the end to life. "I saw you looking at him, girly."

I turned my head, trying not to smile.

He caught me. "I saw you squirming in your seat over there. How wet are those panties?"

I shielded another smile again and said nothing.

He scooted his chair closer to mine and set his hand in my lap. Then, when I didn't argue, he slipped his fingers beneath the waistband of my leggings and the panties underneath. "Very wet," he said.

I said nothing. I watched the fire, and he watched it, too. There, huddled around the orange-and-yellow glow, he slowly stroked my slick wetness over my clit. I put my head against his arm and cried out softly as he increased his speed and I came.

"We'll ask him tomorrow," is what he whispered to me as we climbed into bed that night.

Then he parted my legs, shoved them up high to open my body and drove into me. He fucked me fast and hard until we both climaxed noisily. Then he spooned his warm body against mine, and I fell asleep wondering if Ed would be up for some fun with us in the fucking department.

Dan saw Ed the next morning, and I watched from the dining room as they spoke. I drank my coffee and stared until they got in their separate cars and parted on a wave. It only took a minute or two for my phone to jingle. The text read: *He's coming for dinner. Seven. We'll discuss it then.*

I had a feeling it was going to take a million years for seven o'clock to arrive.

When Dan got home, I had a roast going with potatoes and carrots. A nice bottle of red was open and breathing, and I was in a black dress with silk panties beneath. Dan hooked the hem with a finger and lifted it to peek beneath. He gave a low whistle and said, "Oh, the big guns. Pale turquoise with black lace, and the little lace-up peekaboo thing on the ass."

I waggled my butt at him and laughed. "Only the best when wooing a new one."

"I doubt you'll need to woo," he said, gathering me in his arms. He squeezed me hard and kissed me harder. "But what do I get? Do I get mouth? Pussy? Ass?"

"Be polite and let our guest choose."

He shrugged. "I'll take any of it. Because it's all good." He kissed me again, and that's when the doorbell rang. My blood leapt in my veins, and I smoothed my dress and then my hair.

"Relax, you look great." Then Dan was at the door, ushering in our guest.

I picked at my food, disinterested in meat and potatoes. The men made up for me, though, both going back for seconds. It was over slices of cheesecake that Dan brought up the idea of a threesome.

When he first said it, Ed made him repeat himself. Then he looked at me to see if Dan were somehow joking. I only nodded, trying to smile without fainting. I was nervous. More nervous than usual, in fact.

"If it's a no, we'll understand," I said softly.

"It's not a no. But it's..." He looked at Dan. "This works for you?"

"Has for ten years," Dan said.

"Wow. Um. Sure? Tonight? Is that why you asked me here?"

"We asked you here to get to know you," I said. "Doesn't have to be tonight."

He looked at me, his eyes dipping to the subtle scoop neck of my dress. "Can it be tonight?" he amended quickly.

I glanced at Dan who stood and dropped his napkin. "Damn straight it can be. Wait until you see what's under that dress."

With that, I was led upstairs by my husband, while Ed stayed close on my heels. I felt his eyes on the back of my dress and wondered if he'd like my panties.

He did. He pulled my dress over my head the moment Dan stepped back and leaned against the dresser. When Ed's eyes landed on my panties, he smiled broadly.

"Guest's choice," my husband said, gesturing toward me. Ed understood.

My exposed nipples were erect with want. Ed put his hands on me, pressing his palms to my breasts. He dragged his finger along the cleft of my sex, nudging the soft silk of my undies against my clitoris. I moaned when he lowered his head to kiss my shoulder and then my collarbone.

"If you put your fingers in those panties, I guarantee she's as wet as a waterfall," Dan said softly.

Ed tested his theory. "Very wet," he said.

He tugged my panties down, and my heart fluttered in my chest and I felt a little light-headed. Dan's eyes on us made the moment that much better.

Ed positioned me on my hands and knees on the bed. I readily bent to his will. My new lover ran his fingers along my drenched slit, and then he shoved a finger into me. I bit back a moan, nearly swooning with bliss.

"There are condoms in the nightstand," Dan said.

I was practically vibrating with desire. When Ed rolled the condom on, knelt behind me and slid his cock along my drenched split, I inhaled a shuddery breath. I heard Dan's zipper and then the rustle of his jeans as he stripped them off. He was on the bed with us a moment later, nudging his cock against my lips. I moaned, feeling Ed slip inside my pussy slowly. He was stretching and taxing my body, pushing it to accommodate him. I gasped around Dan's cock, and he groaned, grabbing my hair and tugging my head up so I'd look into his eyes.

He smiled at me, and I sucked him harder, bucking my body back to take Ed's cock. Our neighbor smoothed his hands over my ass, pausing to rotate his hips. His dick was reaching every perfect place inside me; I was hanging there right on the edge of orgasm.

"Make her come," Dan said above me.

Ed began pumping me once more. He gripped one of my hips and then drilled the thumb of his free hand into my asshole as he continued to fuck my pussy.

Caught between the two men—being pushed and pulled deliciously—pleasure coursed through me. Their urgent thrusting took my breath away and caused my heart to bang.

I braced myself with one hand, using the other to stroke my nipples. Then I pinched them hard, until those sparks of pain mingled with the feeling of Ed stretching and filling both of my holes. I came, gagging a bit on Dan's dick.

My husband groaned, driving into my throat a few more times, deep enough to force me to suck in air through my nose. I did my best to keep up, and when he came, I shut my eyes and drank down his load.

Dan backed off, and I bowed down, flattening my upper body to the mattress and moving my ass up higher. Ed's motions increased in intensity, and he pulled his thumb from my back hole only to replace it with a few fingers. The thrusting grew harder and deeper, and I wedged my hand beneath my body to stroke my clit.

"Come for me," he demanded.

I glanced up to see Dan watching us. The sight of him leaning against the wall with a small smirk on his face knocked me over the edge. I stroked my clitoris a little faster, pinched it harder and came, crying out loudly. Ed wasn't far behind me. I felt him pull free of me and heard the snap of the condom. Then he was gracing my back and my ass with hot come.

I started to laugh, even as I tried to catch my breath.

"What's so funny?" he asked as I rolled to my side. He was smiling.

"Nothing," I said. "I was just thinking...welcome to the neighborhood."

His Wanton Wife

SABRINA PORTER

I could tell that Chris was cooking up something the last time we traveled. He'd booked us a room at a nice hotel, probably the nicest we'd ever been in. The bathroom and shower were particularly showy, and he started looking at me oddly the moment I'd commented on it.

I tried to get him to tell me what he was contemplating when we walked on the beach, but he shook his head. I tried again during our dinner at a cozy little crab shack by the water. No such luck. We took a stroll back along the sand and returned to the hotel.

In the elevator, he pushed me to the wall and kissed me. His hands roamed my sides and down my body to cup my ass. When he hauled me close, I felt his hard cock. "I think we need to make sure the sand is washed off you. Really well."

Lust stirred low in my belly, and I nodded. "Yes, okay...yes," I said stupidly. I was so disoriented by arousal that when the elevator stopped, dipping wildly, I cried out.

He caught my wrists up behind my back in one of his large hands. He hustled me to the room and used the key card to open the door. Inside, he pushed me toward the wall with my hands up and my palms pressed to the plain-tan paint job. "Stay," he said.

It never occurred to me to disobey.

I heard the shower come on and then he was back, shoving my short black dress up around my hips. He tugged my panties down until they hugged my knees. Then he pressed himself to the back of me, his cock riding my now-bare asscrack.

"I'm going to stand you in the shower, and you're going to stay where I put you, do you understand?"

"Yes."

"Even when it gets intense, little girl. You hear?"

I could only nod. My pulse pounded heavily in my throat and temples. My pussy seemed to keep the thudding tempo.

Chris dropped to his knees and dragged his teeth along the arch of my right asscheek. Then he dropped gentle kisses along the left. When I was practically shaking with need, he pressed a spit-slickened finger to my asshole and penetrated me. My pussy—empty and eager—clenched tightly around nothing.

I made a sound that was a half laugh, half sob.

Chris stood and lifted my dress over my head before stripping me of my panties. He directed me to kick off my heels, then he led me to the bathroom by my crossed wrists.

"Shut your eyes," he said. "Keep them shut." Without bonds or blindfolds he was dominating—and I was submitting.

I shut my eyes, kept them shut and allowed him to guide me into the tub.

He raised my arms, while using the fingernails of his free hand to scrape across my nipples. Then he kissed me and stroked my clit, making me squirm. I couldn't see what he was doing. Couldn't anticipate what he would do. But my heart thrummed mightily, and I felt light-headed with want.

"Clasp your hands," he said as he placed my wrists on either side of the metal shower curtain bar. I joined my hands as ordered, standing there with my arms up and my pussy wet and wanting.

"Spread your legs," Chris said brusquely. Before he finished the last word, he was knocking my legs wide with his foot. He brushed by me and then he returned. My entire body went rigid when a strong stream of warm water gushed over my pussy.

"I noticed we had a really nice showerhead," he said.

Then his mouth came down on one of my nipples. He bit me in the same spot, and I jumped, my hips shooting forward. The stream of water kissed my clitoris again, and I shuddered. "God," I exclaimed, keeping my eyes shut tight. I wouldn't open them unless he granted me permission.

My shoulders ached and my arms shook from holding the bar, but I wouldn't put my arms down unless he told me to. I was under his command, and that gave me a little thrill.

I heard him click the showerhead setting, and I felt my body sway slightly. The hot water banged against my clit, and as I thrust my hips forward, surrendering to the intensity of the pleasure, he moved the spray once more. The droplets pounded my outer lips and higher, massaging my mound and heating my skin. I whimpered, twisting slightly as I continued to clutch the bar.

"You're doing very well," he said above the hiss of the water. Then it was his mouth that came down on my clitoris.

I almost broke my hold on the shower rod. I forced myself to grip my hands tighter, forced myself to keep my eyes shut. I tried not to lunge toward him for better contact. He held my hips in his hands and sucked the hard knot of flesh. Then his fingers slipped between my legs and into me. Chris worked his thick fingers in and out of me, curved them against the front wall of my cunt, and sucked my clit again.

I gave a soft wail.

"You're only allowed to come from the water," he said. "So hang on, or it will be the last time you climax for a while."

I nodded stupidly. I was desperate to come but also desperate to obey.

His fingers drove in deep, and then he withdrew. When I relaxed, he shoved his digits inside me again. And then he withdrew. Feeling completely off balance and on edge, I tried to breathe deeply.

He chuckled softly at my reactions, and then the water was on me again. The showerhead was on a high setting, the water jetting against my tender flesh. I chewed my lower lip and shivered.

He kissed my upper thighs, angled the water away and then angled the water back. As my body nearly reached its breaking point, he moved the spray once more. I sobbed. This time it was loud—a full-blown sound of need.

Another chuckle came from him, and my nipples pebbled hard and sensitive in the cool bathroom.

"Such a trouper," he said.

Then the spray was back, concentrated right on my pounding clit. The unceasing assault of water on flesh had me trembling.

"You may come, sweetheart."

His words were like magic. He pressed his lips to my hip and moved the showerhead closer to my body, thus increasing the intensity of the water's impact. I came apart at the seams. I climaxed with a loud cry that echoed off the tiled walls of the small room.

"Oh god…oh god." I said it over and over again. I laughed when I said it; I cried when I said it. The orgasm shook me to my core, and I imagined all the things we'd do later in bed.

"Open your eyes," he said.

I looked down at him, and when he nodded, I let go of the bar.

"That was just the appetizer," he said.

"Yeah?" I asked on a shuddery breath.

"Yeah. This hotel room…it inspires me," he said.

"I'm glad," I sighed.

"Really?" He cocked his eyebrow.

I touched his shower-damp hair. "Chris, you have no idea," I said, and wrapped my arms around him.

The Cure for the Common Threeway

Tucker Wallace

My wife, Anastasia, and I have been married for almost ten years. We both have a huge sex drive and screw at least four times a week. She is a blonde-haired vixen with B-cup breasts and a tight pussy and ass. I am a six-foot-tall, blond-haired, blue-eyed man who loves to fuck her sweet cunt and ass as much as I did when we first met.

Recently, we attended a wedding. Since Anastasia was busy being a bridesmaid, I hung out with my buddy, Jasper. At one in the morning, Jasper realized his car had a flat, so Anastasia and I invited him to crash at our house. I promised him I'd help him with the car in the morning. He thought this was a great idea, and we headed home. At our place, Jasper fell asleep on the couch while Anastasia and I retired to our bedroom.

She and I weren't sleepy at all; we wanted to fuck. I took off her dress and licked my way down her body, past her breasts to her smooth pussy. I was about ten minutes into licking her snatch when I felt someone at the doorway. Anastasia and I both looked over to find our naked friend standing there, stroking his cock. It had to be at least eight inches long.

I've known for years that Jasper has wanted to fuck my wife because he and I talk about our sex lives constantly. I knew she wanted to fuck him, too. So I wasn't surprised when my wife beckoned him over and started licking his cock while I continued my pussy eating. After I made her come, she wanted one of us inside her. Jasper positioned her on all fours and slipped his cock into her cunt while I continued to lick her clit. As he worked his cock in and out of her pussy, I kept ringing her clit with my tongue. After about twenty strokes, I found myself making occasional contact with his cock as I lapped at her pussy. This turned me on so much I could not believe it. I was tasting my wife's juices on another man's cock! Anastasia quickly reached another orgasm and decided she wanted to suck that big dick of his.

After several minutes of her giving him head, she directed me to come closer. With Anastasia's encouragement, I leaned in and licked Jasper's cock. We traded his shaft between the two of us, giving him a dual blow job. Jasper put a hand on each of our heads and enjoyed our tongue work. Sharing a man's dick was the most exciting thing that we've ever done. She was deep-throating him while I stroked her hair, and when our friend was ready to come, she released his cock and pointed it at my face. I have never seen someone shoot so much cream. The feeling of him coating my face and coming in my mouth was heaven. And then to have my beautiful wife lick his load off my face and share it with me in an openmouthed kiss was amazing.

We continued our licking and sucking games until the wee hours of the morning. I can't wait to taste another man's come again. Maybe next time I'll even have him fill my ass.

Backdoor Bliss

ERIC WILLIAMS

I don't usually jerk off in public places. Masturbating is something I tend to save for when I am by myself—or ever so occasionally when I'm with my girlfriend. (She does like to stand at my side and watch me manhandle my meat.) But today I couldn't help it. I was checking my mail at my desk when I saw a note from Shoshanna. It wasn't solely an email—it was an email with a video attachment. Sometimes Shoshanna sends me little videos she makes to brighten my day, so I wasn't surprised by the attachment, but I was surprised by what the movie contained.

The video was less than a minute long. In the mini-movie, Shoshanna sat on my bed wearing a harness and a dildo. I could see the football-shaped pillow behind her that she'd given me for my last birthday. I could see that the shades were drawn, and the sunlight through the curtains colored the room with a bluish tint. Shoshanna began stroking her fist up and down her synthetic cock. The thing was fairly realistic in appearance, flesh colored and meant to look like an actual penis. I guess my girlfriend had paid attention when she watched me touch myself. She worked her dick like a pro. The whole time, Shoshanna spoke into the camera, talking directly to me.

"When you get home from work, Eric, this is for you."

That's when I left my desk and went to the men's room. I took the farthest stall in the line, and I brought the phone right up close to my face. I saw the way Shoshanna looked, nearly delirious with plea-sure, as she manhandled her faux dick. "Yeah, baby," she cooed. "I'm going to fuck you tonight, and you're going to love every damn minute."

When the video ended, I played it again. Then again. Then I put the phone in my pocket, and I jacked off. I couldn't stop myself. My breathing was ragged, and I came in what felt like seconds, imagining Shoshanna fucking me the whole time.

We'd never done anything like that before, but we'd talked about it. Shoshanna had even read me a story on pegging that she found in a little book of erotica. But this was new territory. The closest we'd ever come was the time she showed me her vibrator and let me use the device on her. We'd never used any kinds of toys on me.

When I got home that night, Shoshanna was waiting for me. She had on one of my work shirts, buttoned halfway up. I could see the bulge of her synthetic dick pushing out the front of the pale-yellow shirt. I didn't say hello. I didn't ask her how her day had gone. I picked her up and carried her into the bedroom. I tossed her down on my mattress and then got out of my clothes.

Since watching the video, I had thought of nothing else. Now that I was in the presence of the new toy, I had to see the thing for myself.

"Take off your shirt," I told her. My voice was raw with lust. Shoshanna slowly worked the buttons and opened the shirt. Her stunning body was entirely naked except for the harness and the strap-on—the stuff of my fantasies.

I reached forward, about to touch the toy, but Shoshanna playfully slapped my hand away. "You don't touch it with your hand, silly boy," she said. "You suck it with your mouth."

I didn't have a problem with that. I moved closer to her and bent so that I could take her dickhead between my lips. Shoshanna sighed and settled back against the pillows. Her hips began to thrust into the air, so that the dick attached to her harness pushed farther and farther down my throat. I'd never done anything like this before, but the action felt surprisingly natural.

When she had experienced her fill of her first ever blow job, she had me get into position on my hands and knees. I felt the slickness of lube as she oiled up my asshole. Then I felt a brand-new type of twinge as she slid the tip of the cock inside me.

"How do you like that?" Shoshanna asked me, gauging my reaction.

"I like it," I managed to whisper.

"Do you want more?"

"Oh yes," I told her. "Give me more."

Ever so slowly, she slid the cock deeper into my backdoor. I could see her homemade raunchy video in my mind—the way she'd looked, so proud of her new toy. Now that toy was inside me, in a way

I'd never experienced before. Pegging had been a mere wistful dream up until that moment. Shoshanna was making a most treasured fantasy of mine come true.

While she fucked me, she told me how she'd bought the toy on her lunch break the day before. "It was a total whim," she confessed. "I must have walked past that sex toy store hundreds of times without ever going inside. But for some reason, I felt drawn in. I wandered into the place and told the salesgirl exactly what I wanted, and exactly how I wanted to use it."

I choked on a moan. I loved the thought of my darling girl being so bold. I wanted to go with her the next time, so we could buy a different one, maybe even bigger. As if she'd read my thoughts, Shoshanna said, "We'll go together. We'll get one that vibrates next time."

That made me come. I shot hard against the mattress, and Shoshanna immediately pulled out of me and unbuckled the harness and cock. Then she was under me, licking the cream off the tip of my dick, sucking me into her mouth so that I hardly had a chance to go soft. I was erect once more in a heartbeat, and Shoshanna had the lube bottle in her hand.

She looked at me with her brown eyes. I nodded, and she assumed the position. What's good for the gander, in this case, was definitely good for the goose. I oiled up her hole and pressed against her. She started to furiously rub her clit. She hadn't come during our last round, and she was more than primed.

I used my hands to part her perfect cheeks. A quick thrust, and I was in. She started to urge me on under her breath, demanding that I fuck her harder and faster. I did exactly what she said, and a second climax started to build inside me. Shoshanna made herself come with her fast-moving fingertips, and when she reached orgasm, her inner muscles began to squeeze and release. I could feel the contractions in her ass muscles as well, as she milked me to completion. I came with a roar, sealing my body to hers as I emptied my load inside her.

When we were finished, she pulled off and wrapped herself up in a sheet. "You know, now it's your turn," she said. She had an impish look in her eyes.

"For what?" I asked. She couldn't mean anal. I'd just fucked the daylights out of her.

"You make the next movie," she said, "and send it to me at work."

I could feel my breath speed up at the mere thought. Hmm, how would I surprise her? How would I catch her off guard? She'd have to wait and see.

The Office Adonis

TONY ADDARIO

Alexander—otherwise known as the office Adonis—starred in my dreams. Blue eyes. Blond hair. Built like the centerfold of a beefcake magazine, he was the inspiration for every one of my X-rated fantasies.

When Alexander walked past my desk on the way to the copy machine, I sprang an instant hard-on. It's not that he was flirty, or that he said anything seductive, or even that he looked my way. Alexander wears a pair of slacks like nobody's business, and his tight hindquarters in those gray gabardine pants made me want to follow him into the copy room, bend him over the machine and fuck him for hours.

Instead, I focused on the files on my computer screen and prayed for noon to arrive. At lunch, I could retreat to my car, kick back in the seat and jerk off to visions of Alexander blowing me, Alexander offering me his asshole, Alexander being all mine.

When twelve o'clock arrived, I hurried to the garage. My car was parked in the far corner. Thankfully, the place was all but deserted. I practically fell into my seat, my cock as hard as a tire iron. I had been erect all morning. I checked the environment one final time, saw nobody nearby and reclined my seat. I had my dick in my hand, my eyes closed and the radio on, when the passenger door suddenly opened.

"Holy fuck!" I sat up quickly, trying to simultaneously cover myself and make up an excuse for my actions. To my surprise, it was Alexander, who shut the door behind him and looked at me.

"Need help with that?"

I stared at him. Was he offering to *help* me with my erection?

Before I could ask for further explanation, he bent forward and began to suck my dick. Every fantasy I'd ever had about Alexander went streaming through my head: Alexander in the shower. Alexander at the gym. Alexander at my place. Alexander bound and gagged. Nothing compared with the reality of Alexander's pink-lipped mouth as he bobbed up and down on my straining prick.

When I realized that this was real—not another one of my lunchtime masturbatory fantasies—I closed my eyes and relaxed once more. Alexander knew what he was doing. He began to suck harder and move faster as the excitement built inside me. I felt the tightening in my balls, and I gave him fair warning. "I'm going to come," I hissed. Alexander didn't move aside. If anything, he worked me faster and more furiously until I climaxed. He drank every drop of my seed.

I was decimated by the power of my release. Alexander looked at me as he slowly licked his lips. He seemed utterly pleased with himself—the cat that ate the canary. "You're delicious," he said.

"What made you do that?" I had to ask.

"I see the way you look at me. You always stare. But today, you looked as if you wanted to fuck me in half."

"I did," I said. "I mean, I do. Oh fuck, do I want to. I want to take down those nice slacks of yours, lube up your asshole and have at you."

My confession didn't seem to faze him in the slightest. "When?" he asked.

"Right now," I said, but I looked at my watch and realized there was simply no way we could have sex like I wanted and get back to work on time. So I amended my statement. "Tonight. After work. At my place." He smiled at me, and he turned to exit the car. But I wanted more. "Not yet," I said, and there was begging in my voice. "Show me, first."

"Show you what?"

"I want to see where I'm going tonight. Show me."

Alexander gave me a wry little half smile, as if he hadn't expected me to be quite so perverted. Then he unbuckled his belt, undid his fly, and pulled down those glorious slacks. In the tight space of the front seat, he wriggled around to face the window, showing me his haunches encased in a pair of black briefs. I reached forward and pulled the elastic band down, revealing his naked buttocks. Then I parted his cheeks and peered between to gaze at his tight pucker. Dear lord, how I wanted to fuck him right then. But there was no way—not in my car, not on our lunch break.

Because I couldn't help myself, I wet one finger and gently traced the ridge of his asshole. Alexander sighed and bucked at my intrusion. I wanted to rim him. I wanted to nibble around that tight little flower. I reached around and felt his dick. He was hard and leaking precome.

"Tonight," I whispered, "I am going to do such dirty things to you." Then I let him go.

I watched as he fixed his clothes, and then I kissed him. Electricity flowed through me. He gave me a wink before leaving the car, and I knew that all day long I would be consumed by the thought of Alexander's gorgeous asshole.

And I was.

Before six, he stopped by my desk and I wrote down my address. By seven, he was at my place, stripped entirely naked and spread-eagled on my mattress.

Although I'd been a bundle of nervous energy all day long, now I felt calm because I was going to get what I wanted. So I took my time. First, I sucked his beautiful dick. I licked the head as if it were an ice-cream cone. I played with his balls. I stroked his perineum with the tip of my tongue, and he started fisting the sheets and bucking. Only when he was nearly out of his head did I have him roll over while I reached for the lube. Alexander held open his asscheeks for me, and I positively polished his hole with a copious amount of lube.

I got behind him on the bed, and I said, "I'm going to fuck you hard."

Alexander sighed.

"I'm going to fuck you for the way you swish your hips when you walk by my office. I'm going to fuck you for the way you lick your lips when you meet my eyes at meetings. I'm going to fuck you for the way you swallowed my load in the car."

He set his head on the pillow and spread his legs, pulling his cheeks wider apart for me. I pressed the head of my dick to his asshole, and I pushed. Alexander groaned as the first inch of my cock slid inside him. I held him by his hips as I worked him until my cock was entirely buried in his asshole.

Then I began to thrust. Alexander made low humming sounds as I fucked him. I reached beneath him, gripped his cock and began to pump him with my greasy fist. I wanted us to come at the same time, and I teased him with the speed and pressure of my fingers wrapped around his dick while my own cock slid in and out of his hole.

On the cusp, I told him the rest. "We're going to shower," I said, "and then I am going to rim your tight hole. I'm going to make you come with my tongue alone. Then you're going to do the same to me."

Alexander climaxed on my words, and I shot off inside him. I saw shimmering lights behind my shut lids. I saw a galaxy of shooting stars, and then I opened my eyes and saw Alexander, pulling off me, rolling over and gazing up at me. Those blue eyes glowing. That sandy hair falling forward so that he had to do his head tilt to shake the shag out of his way. I bent to kiss him, and we tangled together on the bed and in the sheets.

We didn't have to rush. There was no end to the fantasies we would play out, the ways we would devour each other, the ecstasy that awaited us—my office Adonis and me.

Jessica's Oral Fixation

Patrick Fergusen

When my girlfriend, Jessica, went on her latest diet, I tried to talk her out of it. She's perfect as is, and besides, I've always preferred my women with a little meat on their bones. But Jessica was insistent that she needed to lose a few pounds before serving as maid of honor at her sister's wedding, so I prepared myself for what were sure to be a miserable few months. Nothing good ever comes from Jessica's diets. She spends weeks at a time depriving herself of her favorite treats, and she expects me to do the same in a show of support. Then even if she hasn't ripped my head off out of hunger-induced rage, she's lost some of her soft, sexy curves. Either way, I come out the real loser.

Jessica's newest weight-loss effort came from some kooky blog she'd found online, and she insisted it was a game-changer. I was sure the only game it would be changing was mine, and my ability to get laid until after the wedding, but for once, my girlfriend had found a diet that actually appealed to me.

Jessica printed out the guidelines and hung them on the fridge, but I had no intention of reading them, so she summarized for me. "Basically, it says you have to keep yourself occupied so you don't eat," she told me. "And that means your mouth, too. They suggest drinking lots of water, and if you have to do more, it says you can suck on a lollipop or chew on some ice so you feel like you're eating but aren't actually ingesting more than a few calories." It sounded pretty straight-forward and unimpressive, and I dutifully fixed our icemaker and stocked up on sugar-free lollipops and ice pops.

For a week or so, things went as I expected. Jessica nagged me constantly to "step away from the snack cabinet" and eat healthier treats, and though she seemed to be holding up better than usual, I was getting tired of spending all day listening to her crunch through cups of ice and slurp loudly on her lollipops. Then, her tactics changed.

I was in the bedroom, trying to read a book, when Jessica came in. "I'm sick of ice and candy," she announced. "I looked up what else I could do, and it says I can't chew gum or suck on a mint." There was a strange twinkle in her eye as she said that, and I wondered why she suddenly appeared excited by the idea that she couldn't eat. "I did think of one technique that might be a good substitute," she continued, "but I need your help to test my theory."

I put down my book and stood up, figuring I'd be running to the store to pick up whatever the new miracle snack was, but as soon as I was on my feet, Jessica dropped to her knees in front of me. She pulled down my sweatpants and boxers in one swift jerk, and the next thing I knew, she was fondling my dick as she worked to get me hard.

My cock responded quickly to her touch. Once she had my prick standing at attention, she leaned in and sucked the crown into her mouth. Oh yes! Her tongue swirled around my cockhead a few times before she pulled back and started flicking at the very tip.

She teased me briefly before she sucked me in again, this time pulling me in even deeper. Once she clamped her lips back around my dick, she traced her tongue along the underside. I felt my cock twitch, and I wasn't sure how long I would last. Her oral attention felt too good.

Right when I was starting to think that I was going to come, Jessica pulled back completely. I was startled when I felt cool air hit my dick, and I looked down to see what had caused her to stop. My eyes met Jessica's, and she said, "Mmm, I was right. This is definitely better than sucking on ice cubes."

My cock throbbed at her words. I couldn't speak, but I grunted my agreement and thrust my hips toward her, suggesting she get back to it. She smiled and moved in again, taking my dick into her mouth until my tip touched the back of her throat. I sucked in a breath as she deep-throated me, and when her tongue tickled the base of my cock, I felt my arousal became even greater. Jessica was really giving that blow job her all, and with the way her tongue and lips were moving, and the suction she was applying, I knew there was no chance in hell I'd last much longer. And I didn't care. I wanted to come more than ever before.

My girlfriend started bobbing her head along my length, sucking me from base to tip and back again. The rapid movement and pleasure was enough to set me off, and I groaned loudly as I shot my load straight down her throat.

But the fun wasn't over yet. As soon as Jessica had swallowed every drop of my come, she pulled back, looked up at me and said, "Sweetie, aren't you getting hungry? Do you need me to get you some ice, or maybe…something else?" I knew what she was suggesting, and I was more than game to test out her new method of appetite suppression.

I got down on the floor with her and pushed her onto her back so I could pull off her pants and thong. Then I lay down between her legs and got to work. She was already wet with anticipation, and my tongue moved easily over her slick lips.

I licked around her cunt, cleaning up the juices that clung to her slick flesh, then I started to fuck her with my tongue. I thrust deep into her as she writhed and twisted, her thighs squeezing my head as I hit just the right spot.

Wanting to tease her the way she'd teased me, I pulled back when she started to get really excited and slowly licked around her mound again. I kept up the charade as long as I could, but when she reached down and tried to guide my head back to where she wanted me, I gave in immediately. At the first stroke of my tongue across her hot button, Jessica's pelvis thrust up at my face, and I had to hold her down to stay on target. Once she stilled, I returned to her clit and sucked the nub between my lips. I sucked her and licked her, driving her crazy, and when I felt she was on the verge of orgasm, I nipped at her nub, sending her over the edge.

Afterward, we dressed and went back to what we'd been doing before our brief interlude. But I knew it wouldn't be long before we went for round two. After all, Jessica had a new dress to fit into, and I wanted to be a supportive boyfriend.

Sultry Sex Show

Tawny Webster

Because he knows what gets me off, Joe likes to tie me up on the balcony after dinner. If I get off, he gets off. A happy wife means a happy life.

He used to keep me fully clothed and bind me, leaving me captive as the sun grew dimmer in the sky. The lights from the pool would color me slightly with their aquamarine glow. Then we'd wait. Within moments, the house that was situated across from us would light up. It was the only home within a half mile; a small, grassy field separated us. The neighbor's windows would gradually grow light and then a dark shadow would appear in the upper left window. We assumed it was a bedroom window.

We played this game more and more frequently with the unknown stranger who liked to watch, while we, in turn, liked to show off. A few weeks ago, we amped up the fun. Joe had never fucked me outside before, but he finally did.

After I'd been outside awhile, clothed in a light skirt and blouse, Joe came out and removed my shoes. He placed the shoes on the balcony ledge so they could be seen. Made of thick ornate cinderblocks, the balcony was a sturdy perch for our games.

After twenty minutes or so, Joe came back and removed my skirt. The railing hit me at mid-thigh, so it was obvious, even if viewed from a distance, that I was bare below the waist but for panties. At the point of skirt removal, those panties were soaked in the crotch. When Joe returned to unfasten my blouse, opening it button by button, he stood behind me and reached around to tease my clitoris through my wet panties. His mouth on the back of my neck was hotter than the summer evening. His cock, hard and ready, pressed to the crack of my ass.

I moaned as he left the shirt hanging open. He cupped my left breast with his hand, pinching and tweaking the nipple so that pleasure and pain danced beneath my skin.

I thrust my hips forward against his palm, and then he shoved his hand into my panties, slipping a finger into my cunt. When I sighed, he laughed softly, kissed my neck again and withdrew. Leaving me out there, twisting in the wind, under the watchful eye of our neighbor as warm night air blew across my exposed breasts and raised goose bumps on my skin.

The next time he returned, Joe shimmied me out of my panties, dragging them down slowly so they caressed my thighs and the backs of my knees on the way. The light from the pool appeared brighter and bluer as the sky darkened.

He stood behind me briefly, playing his fingertips across my clitoris, pressing his erection to my bottom. I fought the bonds that held my wrists to the balcony supports.

"What do you want?" His words were hot in my ear.

What did I want? I wanted it all. I wanted everything. But I forced myself to speak words that would make sense. "I want to come."

"Of course, you do."

He dropped down to his knees and moved in front of me. Most likely, to our audience of one, he was nothing but a head that appeared just below my pussy. Joe grabbed my flanks, pushed his face to my sex and slipped his tongue into my wet folds. I bucked my hips forward on instinct, seeking out more contact with his wet mouth. I thrust and my arms twisted, rattling my bonds.

I shivered from the excitement and the sudden warm breeze that washed over me.

Joe got me to the brink—to the sweetest place of all—and then he stood, wiped his mouth, kissed me and left.

Me in my shirt hanging open and unbuttoned and bare everywhere else.

I'm not sure how long I stayed out there like that, exposed but for the fluttering of my top around my shoulders to the shadow in the window across the way. When he returned, Joe gathered my long hair in his hand and wrapped it once around his fist. He tugged lightly before scraping his teeth along the back of my neck until I moaned, my nipples hardening instantly.

"Is he there?"

Joe knew the answer, but he wanted me to say it. "He's there."

"Is he watching my pretty, pretty girl?"

I whimpered as he once more ground his cock against my ass. I wanted him in me. I wanted him to fuck me. I wanted the grand finale, and yet I didn't want it to end. My pulse pounded in my temples, my throat—my pussy. Joe had teased me by taking me right to the brink, and I was still there. Wet and ready and desperate beyond measure.

His fingers played across my nether lips. He teased my clit and slid a digit inside me. "Answer me."

"He's watching me."

"Nope."

I almost laughed, but he had me too worked up. "He's watching your pretty, pretty girl?"

"Good." He angled me forward, pulling my feet back a little until I was exactly the way he wanted. I knew the pool light shined on the balcony and illuminated it. I knew that we could be seen, almost as if we were spotlit. I knew all this, so when I heard Joe's zipper go down I almost came from the sound of it. I heard his pants hit the deck and his belt buckle jingle. I heard the whoosh of his shirt coming off.

My nipples stood out—hard ready peaks—and my stomach dipped as if I were riding a roller coaster.

Joe's hands gripped my hips, and his cock nudged me. I pushed my ass out and let him get to the exact spot he needed. He thrust slowly but firmly, and then I gasped because he was in.

I was so wet, so ready, it took no time to work up to a crazy rhythm. He drove into me, lifting me up on my tippy-toes, straining my arms in their bonds so they ached. But the ache only added to the rush of pleasure I was feeling from our fucking.

I hung my head, hoping our viewer could see how utterly perfect this all was. My hair curtained me from looking, but I swore I could feel the stranger's eyes on me. More than once we'd thought we'd seen the subtle flash of lenses reflecting light as if our neighbor had binoculars. I could only hope he did.

I pushed back to take Joe, slamming my body to meet every lusty thrust. He began to make soft, deep noises. I stared at his bare feet between my legs, trying to focus my attention so that I didn't climax too soon. I could tell he was close, and I wanted more than anything to come with him. One big finale for the appreciative man across the way.

But Joe played dirty. He reached around and found my clit, slippery with my own juices, and began to rub firm circles on top of that swollen knot as he continued to pound me. Within moments, I was coming, crying out into the night as my hair swayed before my face and my calf muscles screamed from the tension of holding myself in position.

I felt him pull free of me so quickly that I gasped. Joe came around to my side, his fist working his cock furiously. "Just to keep things interesting," he whispered, pressing close as he climaxed. His come splashed my thigh and my belly. His breath was loud and ragged in my ear.

I let my head fall back as I moaned because the warm splash of his cream added a whole new layer of dirty to this game.

"Next week—"

"Next week, I'll come on something else," he said, grinning. "We have all week to work it out. I'm sure he'll appreciate the visual."

I nodded. Then I laughed, because I knew as soon as he undid my bonds, I'd be using my shaking hands to get myself off again. His moment of inspiration had put me back to the beginning. Ready to come. Desperate to get off.

His Straying Spouse

KEVIN POTTER

I knew Cindy was sleeping around on me. As much as my wife liked to think she could keep a secret, she had a terrible poker face. I quickly figured out what she was up to—and it changed my life in a completely unexpected way.

I'd been suspicious since she'd mentioned wanting to host a ladies-only card game at our house on the nights I played basketball with the guys. In ten years of marriage, I'd never seen my wife play so much as a game of solitaire, but at first I assumed she was making up an excuse to get together with her girlfriends to gossip—her favorite pastime. The first few weeks, I noticed that the fridge seemed well stocked after her game nights. I assumed she and her friends were mostly drinking wine or had ordered takeout. After a few weeks of this,

I decided to go on the hunt in our home for playing cards. I couldn't remember the last time I'd come across any in the house, and after scouring the place from top to bottom, I discovered that we didn't own a single deck.

By then, I was really curious, so when my weekly basketball game was canceled, I kept the change of plans a secret and decided to see what my wife was really doing. I left the house like usual on Thursday night and drove around the block. I stopped at the local fast-food place and grabbed a burger and fries, and once I'd eaten, I figured enough time had passed that I could sneak back to the house. I parked down the street and walked home through the neighbors' backyards. When I got close enough, I saw a strange car in our driveway, but only the one. Most of my wife's friends are soccer moms who drive large SUVs.

I needed to get closer, so I walked around the house and peeked in each window I passed until I found what I was looking for. I was standing in front of the living-room window, through which I saw Cindy on her knees, naked, sucking some guy's cock. I didn't know the man, but he was definitely my wife's type: tall and muscular and fair. I wondered where she'd met him and how this had all started. I decided to watch for a minute, wanting to know more about this affair she was having before I stormed in and confronted her.

Something happened as I watched, though. After a couple minutes, instead of being angry, I was aroused. I no longer wanted to confront my wife; I wanted to join her. I'd never imagined opening my marriage or even cheating, but there was something incredibly hot about seeing my wife in action with another man. My arousal surprised me, but as my cock throbbed in my pants, I knew I couldn't deny how excited I was.

Cindy and I have never had bad sex, and even at our busiest, we still get it on at least four times a week, so I couldn't imagine she wasn't satisfied. But we'd been college sweethearts, and neither one of us had had much experience when we got together. I know I'd wondered about what else was out there, and I guess my wife had, too. Unlike me, however, she'd decided to find out what she was missing.

My eyes were glued to my wife as she released the man's cock from her mouth, turned around and sat down on his lap, impaling herself on his shiny shaft. Then she started riding him. I'd never seen my wife like that before. We'd never fucked in front of a mirror or filmed ourselves, so I'd only ever seen her up close. Watching her whole body writhe and seeing the expressions she made was one of the most arousing experiences of my life.

I was getting more and more excited as I watched them. I wanted to jerk off, but I was afraid of getting caught with my pants down, literally. Meanwhile, inside my house my wife was getting what looked like incredible pleasure. Now, instead of being upset, I was jealous. I envied her for being able to get off when I couldn't, and I envied her date for getting to experience my wife at her most wanton. I was very tempted to run in and break up their party so I could fuck her instead, but I didn't want to give up the sexy show, so I stayed put and continued to observe.

The guy was really getting into it as Cindy rode his cock, and he reached one arm around her so he could fondle her breasts, while his other hand slipped south to toggle her clit. When he touched her button, she turned her head toward him, and after sharing a deep kiss, she leaned back and started thrusting even harder. Her back arched and her breasts jutted out, and then she seemed to get even more into the fucking. She started swirling her hips and shifting side to side, and I knew from experience exactly how good that felt.

I sensed Cindy's orgasm coming on, and I was excited to see her climax. I kept my eyes on her face as she got closer and closer, and when her orgasm hit, her eyes slammed shut and she bit her lip. Her partner must have come, too, because I saw his muscular body tense beneath hers.

I continued looking on as the couple before me parted and the guy got dressed and headed for the door. As soon as he was gone, I hurried back to get my car and drove home again. Cindy wasn't expecting me to return so early, and her surprise was evident when I walked in the door only minutes after her secret lover had exited. But I needed to get off, and I couldn't wait another minute to get my hands on her—and my cock in her.

I grabbed Cindy as soon as I saw her and planted the most passionate kiss on her lips. That, too, seemed to surprise her, but she was obviously still aroused, because she returned the kiss with equal passion. I guided her over to the couch and quickly pulled her panties off from under her skirt before pushing her over the arm. Then I pushed down my shorts and guided my already rock-hard cock into her still-dripping slit. I fucked her as hard and as fast as I could, desperate for release after watching her with her boyfriend. She responded quickly, thrusting her ass back to meet my strokes, and I felt my cock throb rapidly as I neared climax.

I'd never come so fast in my life. I'd barely been fucking Cindy for two minutes before I couldn't hold back any longer. When it became impossible to hold on, I totally let go, filling her with my seed. But I didn't stop pounding her until she climaxed—again.

I've never told Cindy that I found out about her affair, but I did start skipping my basketball games regularly so I could watch her get it on with her lover. Her screwing around has been the best thing to happen to our sex life yet!

Spanking Good Fun

Jackie Martise

My husband likes to surprise me with new playthings. Recently, Will spilled his potato chips all over the floor and then asked me if I'd mind grabbing the broom. Tucked inside the closet, in front of the broom and the mop, was a riding crop.

As I stood, gaping, he came up behind me, gripped my hips and rubbed himself against me. "I bought it yesterday. I thought we'd take advantage of having the house to ourselves today."

He took my long blonde braid in his hand and tugged gently. "Bring it to the living room, so we can give it a go." He led me by my hair as I tried to focus on him and the crop—and not the pounding of desire in my cunt. "How about if you get on the ottoman?" he asked, tapping the back of my leg with the leather tip of the crop. As he pulled the implement back, I noticed the keeper was in the shape of a hand. A jaunty little leather hand just over the moon about smacking red marks up the backs of my thighs, along my flanks and across my ass.

I draped myself over the ottoman, my belly flat against its top. My head hung over one side, my vulnerable ass at the other. He hiked up my denim skirt and started dragging the tip of the crop over the soft silk of my panties.

"Mmm," he said. "I like these. These are soft. And very orange."

I chuckled. They were *very* orange. I'd bought them on my last lingerie-shopping trip. I'd been amused by their brightness. I'd bought two similar pairs in shocking yellow and bright magenta. The colors reminded me of sherbet.

My laugh wasn't welcome, though; it earned me a good, quick blow from the crop. I yelped, my body bowing, my head flying back. My braid, thick and smooth, slid across my back.

"Focus on what we're doing," he said.

"Yes, Will," I responded breathlessly, but it was difficult for me.

I could feel a craving deep inside me, the wet, greedy pound of need in my pussy. My clit thrummed as if electric currents were moving across my flesh. I prayed for him to touch me, Christ, anywhere—even the soles of my feet. I felt as if stimulation *anywhere* would bring me to orgasm.

"Your mind's wandering," he said, and the crop came down across the meatiest part of my bottom. The blow stung both asscheeks and settled deep in my slit. I clenched my internal muscles to eke out some pleasure, which was cheating, and I knew it. Will caught me, like he always does. Three fast blows landed against the backs of my thighs. Arousal beat insanely beneath my skin.

I hung my head and longed for a finger, a tongue, a cock—anything to satisfy my hunger.

"You're free to beg off. Just say the word, and I'll stop," he said, squatting down to talk right into my ear.

I shook my head, braid flying. I'd say my safeword when hell froze over. All the heady discomfort he delivered morphed quickly into an addictive pleasure that my whole body seemed to reach for.

I pushed my ass back, and his hand moved to slide gently along the swell of each buttock. Will traced his finger down the crack of my ass, pausing to press a fingertip to my asshole through my panties. Then he scooted the panties down slowly, so I could feel the glide of luxurious fabric over crop-warmed skin.

"Now be a good girl..." He went for the left first. The pain was smart and fast. Before I could recover, he'd moved to the right. I felt heat blossom in my skin, and I wiggled because somehow it was easy to think in that moment that if I moved the crop would hurt less.

Not true.

Side to side, he alternated, not too hard but definitely not soft. Will whipped me until I was practically fucking the ottoman. Sobs and moans slipped out of me, and when he stopped, I inhaled a great, shuddery breath.

His fingers drove into me, and I almost came. I bit my lip to hang on. I counted in my head. I prayed. Then I felt him get down behind me. He blew softly against me from behind. Coolness erupted along my nether lips; my clitoris seemed to pulse.

"Help me," I managed to utter.

He knew what I meant. His zipper sounded immensely loud in the small room as he lowered his fly. His cock dragged along my soaking-wet split, teasing me. He dragged it down to kiss my clitoris, the tip wet with my juices. He brought me to my first orgasm that way, stroking my clit with his smooth cockhead.

I shuddered, able to breathe again.

"Please," I gasped, one last shuddery plea.

And then he was in me, sliding one arm beneath my belly, holding me to him while driving deep inside me. He bucked his hips, and my body arched in response. I moved back to take him. I met every thrust with eager abandon. And finally, I put my head down and let him hold me and take me.

I came again, my body gripping tight around his pistoning cock. When he withdrew, I shivered. But I knew what was coming from our previous play sessions, and excitement unfurled in me.

Will moved to the front of the ottoman and jammed his cock—wet from my cunt—into my mouth. From his new position, he was able to fuck my mouth while smacking my ass with the crop. When I sucked deep, the blows were lighter; when I backed off, the blows were harder. I kept him off balance as much as I was able, until he grunted, "You're a slutty girl. I shouldn't reward you. But touch yourself. I want you to come with me."

It was a magical moment of synchronicity. He drove into my mouth as I sucked him off, my fingers sliding—slippery and shaky—over my clit, the crop keeping time on my flesh.

When he broke our rhythm and came, painting my lips and chin with his cream, I climaxed. My mouth popped open, and I tasted the last drops of him on my tongue.

He stroked my cheek and bent down to kiss me, which turned me on all over again. "I have bad news," he said.

"What?"

"We still need that broom," Will said, laughing.

I nodded. "Well worth it," I whispered, still trying to catch my breath. "Well, well worth it."

Taking the Temp

Benjamin Houston

The first time I met Danny I knew he was the third we'd been looking for. He came in as an IT temp when our regular guy went out for a few weeks to spend time with his new wife on their honeymoon. Danny was tall, buff and blond. He was funny but sort of quiet. It only took one conversation with him to know my Natalie would love him.

She'd love him even more in our bed.

I took him to lunch once. Then I asked him to meet up with the rest of us after work for a beer. Then I asked him out for a beer alone. And finally, I dropped the bomb when I felt we'd gotten to know each other fairly well.

It was over another beer at the pub near the office.

"You know, Nat and I would love to have you over for dinner one night," I said.

"Sure, that'd be great."

"We'd also love for you to be our third some night."

It took him a moment to understand what I was proposing, and that was the moment where I found myself holding my breath. Usually, this step went fairly well. A few times in the past it had gone awry. When he spoke, he asked if I'd get jealous. I assured him that I wouldn't, that seeing my wife with him would be a huge turn-on and that I liked and trusted him.

After finishing his beer, he agreed.

I invited him over for dinner the next night and called Nat. She'd been beyond excited. It was all I could do to keep her satisfied until the following evening came.

Danny showed up wearing jeans, a polo shirt and a pair of sneakers. We shook hands, and I noticed he was a strange mix of extremely confident and obviously nervous.

Nat kissed his cheek at the door, which he seemed to find endearing. She wore a red sundress and silver sandals, and her long brown hair was swinging wild. We ate burgers and drank beers on the patio. I kept my conversation to a minimum to let them get to know each other. After dinner we moved inside, and that's when Natalie— my wild child—unzipped her dress, stepped out of it, and dropped it in Danny's lap as she said, "Dessert's in the bedroom, boys."

Then she sauntered up the steps, taking her time, bare-assed naked. I watched Danny try not to goggle at her.

"It's hard," I said. "And I live with her."

"Hard to what?" he asked after a long pause where he seemed

to be trying to gather his thoughts.

"Hard not to stare. Hard not to want."

"I still can't believe you invited me here," he said.

"I did. And I invited you here for that," I said, pointing toward the stairs. "More than the beer and burger."

"So..."

"So we should get up there," I said.

He stood so fast he almost lost his balance. "And we...me and you?" He let the question hang.

I laughed. "Some contact is usually unavoidable. Beyond that, I'm open, but it's not obligatory. It's basically whatever you're comfortable with."

Danny seemed okay with that because he gave me a nod, set his beer down and took the stairs two at a time. I was right behind him.

In the bedroom, Natalie was lying across our bed, legs spread and fingers playing slowly over her pussy lips. When we both entered, she found her clit with her fingertip and gave herself a slow, even stroke. "I was starting to worry," she said with a mock pout.

Danny's eyes slid to me, and I grinned. "Go on," I said. "Don't keep the lady waiting."

"What..." He looked uncertain but then finished his query. "What do you want?"

"For you to take off those clothes, stud," Natalie said. She winked at me.

I took off my shirt but waited on the pants. When Danny began to unfasten his belt buckle, Natalie looked ready to come right there.

"Easy, girl." I chuckled.

"He's perfect," she said to me.

"I thought you'd like him," I said.

When Danny was naked, she curled a finger at him. "Come on. Let's get better acquainted."

Danny climbed onto the bed, and I took off my pants. Natalie was kissing him, stroking his cock with her hand so he grew harder. She motioned for him to move up and straddle her chest, and when he did, she took his cock in her mouth. She sucked him hard, and I found myself holding my breath.

Seeing her for the first time with a new lover is always a treat.

I moved to the bed but didn't get on, giving them a moment first. When Danny was thrusting in and out of Nat's mouth and panting, I sat on the bed and pushed my fingers deep inside her pussy. She was slick and perfect around my fingers. I added a third digit and nudged her G-spot until she was raising her hips and mewling around his pistoning dick. I rubbed my thumb against her swollen clit and jammed my fingers deep again.

She came, lapping at Danny eagerly before breaking their connection in order to catch her breath.

"I want him in my pussy," she said to me.

I moved away to let Danny position himself between her parted thighs. He smiled broadly at me, which let me know he was comfortable. I handed him a condom, and Natalie sat up to roll it on him. She did it like a pro, and he hummed as she finished. When he slid into her, she gave a cute little squeal. She hooked her legs behind his back and moved in time with his eager movements. After a beat she turned to me and said, "What are you waiting for, baby?"

She didn't have to ask me twice. I slipped my cock between her lips, where our guest had been only minutes before. I pulled out, sank a bit lower and shut my eyes as she sucked my balls and then licked them gently. Then I plunged my dick into the wetness of her mouth. She likes to almost gag on me, and I never argue.

I fucked her mouth as Danny took his time screwing her cunt. Her hands gripped his arms, and she jerked so furiously that her breasts bounced in time with her movements. Danny lowered his head to suck her nipple into his mouth. When he used his teeth on her nub, she came as her mouth clamped down around my pumping cock.

"Fuck," I said through gritted teeth.

Danny nodded. "I know."

"Roll over, Nat," I snarled.

We both moved back, and she rolled onto her hands and knees. I pushed between her lips, feeling the scrape of her teeth. I liked it. She switched speeds to suck my balls again. When Danny moved to slide into her, she said casually, "How about in the ass, big boy?"

He froze, and then looked at me for confirmation. "She means it," I said. "Go on."

"Lube?"

"You're wet enough," Natalie sighed.

Her juices had liberally slickened the condom, and after one more glance my way, he parted her asscheeks and began to ease his way in. Her mouth on me was chaos—licking, sucking, lapping—and I had to focus hard on not coming.

When he was in, he shuddered. I knew it wouldn't be long at all, maybe three or four good strokes. Her fingers were working her pussy, and her mouth was making me very happy. I bit my lip to hold on. Danny gripped her hips so tightly her skin blanched white.

He drove into her as she moaned around my cock. I held her

head, he held her ass and then he slid deep, rocking her forward, and hissed, "Jesus Christ."

He pulled free, whipped the condom off and came all over her ass. His come striped her tan skin pearly white.

She moaned around me again, and I knew she'd made herself climax. When she looked up at me with those big blue eyes and shuddered from her orgasm, I let go and shot into her mouth. She swallowed my load as the climactic spasms grew softer and farther apart.

Then she pulled back and smiled. "I like your new friend."

"Me too."

"Will you come back?" she asked Danny, rolling onto her back.

"As often as you like," he replied.

Danny doesn't temp for my company anymore, but he's still a regular visitor to our house.

Meeting Her Match

Jewel Rodriguez

Weddings turn me on. I didn't realize this right away. What happened was that I started being asked to participate in my sorority sisters' weddings. There were so many, one after the other. I experienced countless fittings for the pretty, pastel chiffon dresses. I attended engagement parties on yachts, in parks, even at a bowling alley. I drank more champagne than anyone has a right to. At some point, while one of my fellow "sisters" confessed that she dreaded yet another extravaganza, I realized how much I loved every moment.

Maybe that's because I always managed to hook up with a hot groomsman. I had a knack, I suppose, of picking the perfect single friend of the groom to pay attention to. By the day of the event, I'd have my chosen man wrapped around my finger and raring to go. Then all

I had to do was wait for the proper moment—generally right after the nuptials—to pounce. I'd snag my groomsman, and we'd go at it at in an alcove, or a limo, or out behind the hall. I was not particular as long as I got to say, "Oh yes," after the bride said, "I do."

Last Saturday was my twelfth time as a bridesmaid. I made eyes at Gregory the whole week leading up to the big day. I danced extra close to him at the Jack-and-Jill bachelorette party. I stroked him under the table during the rehearsal dinner. On the morning of the wedding, I was surprised to find him outside my hotel room door.

"What are you doing here?" I asked, confused.

"Don't tell me it's bad luck," he teased. "You're not the bride."

I was already in my melon-colored chiffon strapless gown. Gregory had on his sleek gray suit. Of all the men I'd met at weddings, he was by far my favorite. He had a dirty sense of humor, a sly way of looking at me to make sure I'd gotten his double entendres. I liked his style, and his charming attitude with the rest of the guests—with that special sexual undercurrent he seemed to save for me. But I hadn't expected this situation. This was the first time one of my flirtations had gotten out of hand. I'd always been the one in charge, but not now.

He backed me into the room, and said, "Take that off. You won't want to rumple it."

I didn't say no, because the sight of him had made my panties wet. I didn't say anything except, "We have to be at the church in less than an hour."

"Then we'll have to hurry." He was in motion, carefully pulling my dress over my head, pawing at my undergarments. I'd been imagining our impending tryst, so when he reached into my panties, he found that I was positively drenched.

"Weddings turn you on," he said, and he wasn't asking, but I nodded as I dropped to my knees. He undid his fly and released his thick, fat cock. I started to suck him, thinking about how in less than sixty minutes I'd be standing across from him, looking as sweet and innocent as ever. That made me work him extra hard, and he moaned and braced himself with his hands on my shoulders.

"Tell me why?" he queried, but how could I with my mouth full of his cock? He seemed to understand my predicament, because he pushed me back and then had me get on the bed. In seconds, he was between my legs, pulling off my panties and starting to go down on me. "Tell me," he insisted in between licks of his tongue against my juicy snatch. "What's the big turn-on?"

I didn't know what to say. Nobody had ever figured me out before. How had Gregory guessed that I was a wedding slut? I managed to murmur, "I like the pomp and circumstance. All the preparations feel like foreplay to me."

He pinched my clit as a reward for my confession, and then he drew hard on that swollen button and made me come. I shivered on the bed, lost in the bliss he was creating for me with his magic mouth. While the sweet contractions were still pulsating through me, Gregory rolled me over and got me on my hands and knees. I felt the fabric of his slacks against me as he prepared to fuck me doggie-style.

"How many weddings have you been to?" he asked.

"I've been a bridesmaid in twelve," I panted. His cock was long and thick, and he managed to hit me in all the right places. I wondered how many times he would make me come before we had to sprint to the church. He knew exactly how to take me. He drove his cock into my pussy, and he ran one hand under my body to lightly stimulate my clit at the same time. I rested on my elbows, pushing my ass higher in the air as he rammed me. He timed our orgasms precisely, rubbing my clitoris harder as he fucked me faster. In what felt like seconds, I was coming again, and this time, Gregory climaxed with me. I felt him shooting deep inside me, and then he pulled out and I whipped around, slurping all my copious juices off his cock.

He hadn't expected that, and he groaned as I licked him. I was so turned on by his surprise visit that I made it my mission to get him hard once more. It didn't take long. When he was ready again, his dick as hard as steel, I told him to get out of his clothes. He stripped quickly, and then I pushed him onto the bed so he was on his back. I climbed astride him and began to bounce up and down on his dick. He palmed my breasts and told me how pretty I looked, how he'd been raring to fuck me from the first time he'd caught sight of me.

"And then when I realized you liked weddings…" he said.

"How did you know?"

"You just lit up every time anyone talked about the ceremony, the dinner, the limo…most guests glazed over, but you hung on every detail."

"Speaking of hung…" I grinned at him. I loved the way his big dick felt inside me. When he reached for me and pulled me toward him, I was rewarded with the dulcet sensation of his mouth kissing and licking first one nipple, then the other.

I came, grinding my hips against his, moaning with the ecstasy that flooded through me. He pulled out and flipped me around, and this time, he gave me a pearl necklace, shooting all over my chest and tits.

"I have to go to a wedding next weekend," he said as we showered together, noting the fact that we were due to the chapel in only minutes. I could feel the tingles start at my toes and begin to work up my body. "Would you be interested in being my date?"

"Oh, yes," I sighed with heartfelt enthusiasm.

"In fact," he said, "three of my frat brothers are getting married this summer. Maybe you'd like to be my date for all of the weddings."

"I do!" I told him. "I mean, I would."

"But you can't fuck another groomsman," he said, "only me."

I was fine with that, so fine.

Now I've found a groomsman who loves weddings as much as I do. And who knows? Maybe someday the wedding we fuck at will be our own!

The Bling's the Thing

Stella Piazza

For New Year's, I go all out. I like baubles, bangles, tiny white lights dangling from every nook and cranny. Peter indulges my whims because he doesn't mind a little glitter if the mood is bright. But this year, I wanted to go further. Not only did I deck the halls and the stairwell and the bedroom (as well as the car, our home office, and the tiny patio outside the kitchen)—I also decked myself. I'd read about the concept of bejeweling one's privates online. The official term for the procedure is *vajazzling*, and I was intrigued. I'd even watched a video that showed exactly how clever the nether artist could be.

What would Peter think if I adorned my area down there? I wasn't sure, but I decided to find out. He's always been supportive of my various style whims. When I shaved my pubes into a heart, he was charmed. When I went with a landing strip of fur, he dove right in. Now, I was going to be totally bare, but blinged to the max, and I couldn't wait. I booked an appointment so that when Peter lifted my dress on New Year's Eve, I would sparkle from head to toe—and especially in the middle! I'll admit to being a little nervous. I've never been the type of girl to follow every fad—and this one was definitely among the more unusual. However, the thought of surprising Peter in this way made me swallow my nerves and keep the appointment.

The technician was adorable and funny, putting me quickly at ease and suggesting different designs I might try. I already knew what I wanted—a star. Wouldn't that be perfect for New Year's? And besides, it's Peter's nickname for me because my name means Star in Latin (and French and Greek).

Once I had myself all jeweled up, I could hardly wait for the big reveal. I wanted to go right home, rip off my clothes and show Peter what I'd done. It took every ounce of my willpower not to do exactly that, but Peter had planned a big night for us. I didn't want to steal the show.

That night, we both dressed up. Peter looked stunning in his tuxedo. I put on a cocktail dress that was woven through with silver threads. The hem came barely to my upper thighs. I didn't wear panties, and I was conscious all evening of the gems adorning my pussy. We went to dinner at a fancy club. There was dancing afterward, and I kept telling myself to be patient. My time would come. However, when Peter suggested a moonlit walk along the pier, I put my foot down.

"No, we have to go home!"

"It's not even eleven yet, Stella," he said, surprised by my reaction.

"Home!" I insisted.

He agreed, yet he was clearly confused by my attitude. I let him be until we walked in the door of our apartment. It was decked in glitter, as always for the holiday. That was no surprise to Peter. What was a surprise was when I whipped off my little shimmery cocktail dress and cocked a hip at him.

"Oh, my," he said, the lights glinting off my sparkling self. "What did you go and do, Star?"

He went on his knees for a closer look, and I leaned against the wall of the hallway and spread my legs. His fingertips danced lightly over the gems. He seemed afraid to touch, but he was quite clearly lost in admiration.

"You're a true star now," he said, and I smiled down at him. "Literally," he added, his fingers making another trip up and over the tiny shining jewels. Carefully, cautiously, he parted the lips of my pussy and began to tease me with his tongue. I hadn't actually thought about the next step—what would happen after I'd made the reveal. I'd been so excited simply to show off my sparkly self that I hadn't bothered to mentally play out the rest of the evening's events. Peter knew what to do. He licked and kissed my pussy, being very careful not to stir my gems. Every few laps, he settled back on his knees and admired me some more. He seemed to genuinely appreciate the trouble I'd gone to in setting up this display.

"When did you do this?" he asked during one of his pauses.

"This afternoon. It's been torture not to show you!"

"Let me reward you," he said, and he started to spiral around my clit the way that always gets me off. I groaned and bucked my hips forward, lost in the sweet haze of pleasure that Peter created. I called out his name as I came on the tip of his tongue, and then I slid down the wall until we were face-to-face. He kissed me, and I tasted my own essence on his tongue. I reached forward and felt how hard he was. Would he fuck me there, on our polished floor? Would he take me to the living room, with the lights strung on the mantel? No, he carried me to the bedroom. With the overhead lights out, but the magical fairy lights on, our room seemed to glow like a mystical wonderland. The lights even caught the diamond-like gems on my skin, and Peter was mesmerized.

"You always add sparkle to any room," my man said to me as he got between my legs once more. "But now, you even sparkled your pussy."

I laughed as Peter softly stroked me. I could tell that he was gearing up to fuck me into the New Year. But he didn't seem to want to stop in his appreciation for my private parts. He kept moving into new angles so that he could see the light shine on the jewels.

"You're so beautiful," he sighed, his fingertips taking another leisurely trip around the sparkling star shape adorning my pussy. "I could stare at you for hours. But I want to fuck you, too."

He licked my slick split again, taking me almost to another orgasm before I demanded that he enter me. I needed to feel his cock.

"Is it okay?" he asked. "Will the jewels stay on?"

I nodded enthusiastically. The technician had assured me that the body glue would last through a lovemaking session. In fact, she guaranteed that not a jewel would fall off for several days. Peter stripped and got back on the bed. He entered me sitting up, pushing my knees up toward my shoulders, so he could keep admiring my pretty pussy while we fucked.

"I don't know how you kept that a secret all night," he said breathlessly as he plunged inside the wet heat of my pussy.

"It wasn't easy," I confessed. "I wanted to flash you at dinner. I wanted to pull up my dress on the dance floor."

"Next time," he said, and I realized he liked the special decorations on my private parts so much that there would be a next time. *Maybe Valentine's Day*, I thought, already planning the shining ruby heart I'd request for the love of my life.

Pretty Panties

Melanie Klein

Len is aware of my fixation with pretty panties. Even so, when he sent me an email while I was at work, I wasn't expecting to see an attached photo that showed a gorgeous pink-and-black shopping bag. A bag from my favorite lingerie shop.

The sight turned me on almost instantly, and I actually reached out and stroked the picture on the screen. I shot back an email asking what time he'd be home.

When he told me four, I glanced at the clock. I only had three hours to wait, but those three hours took forever.

At home, I rushed inside the house to find the downstairs silent and the shades still drawn. But Len's keys were on the table and his truck had been out front, so I knew he—and my prize—were there.

I dropped my bags and rushed up the steps to find him sitting in the chair at the foot of our bed. He had his legs crossed, an ankle resting on his opposite knee as he impatiently jiggled his work-booted foot. When he saw me, his blank look turned into a wolfish grin.

"There she is. Ready for your surprise, baby?"

I was so out of breath and so far past turned on, I could only nod.

Len tossed the bag on the bed where it landed with barely a sound. Whatever was inside wasn't heavy enough to cause much noise at all. But before I took a step, he twirled a finger in my direction. "Go on. Take it all off."

Mindless with lust, I kicked off my heels and removed my dress. Beneath I wore dove-gray panties and a matching bra. Gifts from him not too long ago. He smiled again. "Nice panties. But let's get rid of those, and see what's in the bag."

Then he clapped once smartly, and as if on command my pussy flexed, wet and eager, and I unhooked my bra. I shoved my panties down and had to force myself to take a deep breath. I moved to the bed, supremely aware of his eyes on my naked body as I walked.

"It is almost a shame to cover up that ass with panties. But I buy them for you because you get so very wet when I do. Wet and slick and downright filthy."

His wicked chuckle tickled my spine, and I shivered. I opened the bag and parted the black tissue paper, my body humming with anticipation. They were folded with great care. Delicate little things. Pale, pale yellow. Silk panties—tanga cut—and a demi-cup bra. I realized I was holding my breath only when tiny spots of white light appeared in my vision.

I inhaled deeply and pulled the dainty garments from the bag. I put the bra on the bed and stepped into the panties. They were so soft that the feel of them sliding up my thighs caused my nipples to spike quickly.

"I see you like them," Len said. His eyes were pointedly aimed at my breasts. The weight of his gaze coupled with the feel of new lingerie caused goose bumps to race across my skin. After another shiver, I put on the demi-cup bra. The shallow cups barely covered my nipples—nipples that had become so sensitive that when the fabric touched them, my pussy grew wet and I felt my new panties getting seriously damp.

Len flicked a finger toward the bed. "Get up there and show me how much you like your presents."

I stretched out on the bed, facing him. I spread my legs and began to stroke my clit through my luxurious new panties. I felt the crotch grow damper still as Len unzipped his pants and pulled his thick, hard cock free. He began to stroke himself in time with my self-love. I raised my hips, driving my hardened clit against my fingers. I pushed down one of the barely there demi cups and teased my nipple before pinching it hard.

A moan slipped out of me, and Len made a gruff sound in response.

I rubbed myself harder, driving the delicate fabric against my own delicate spot, while moving my free hand to the other nipple. I slipped my finger along my silk-covered slit before returning to rub my clitoris roughly.

"I want you to come so I can fuck you," he said. "I know you're wet inside those panties. But I want you drenched. I want the crotch of these knickers to be sopping."

I sighed, my eyes drifting shut as I pinched the tight knot of my clit before rubbing it more vigorously.

"Look at me," Len said.

I opened my eyes and stared at him. He stroked his cock slowly, but I could tell his grip was tight. At the top of every stroke, he thumbed the head of his prick, spreading precome around the tip. I licked my lips, rubbed a bit harder, and when he cradled his balls in his free hand, I found myself coming as if he'd touched me instead of himself.

He stood fast, approached me faster, and then the bed dipped with his weight. Len pushed himself between my legs and began to grind his hard cock against the wet crotch of my panties.

"You like these?" he said in a raspy voice filled with want.

I could only nod.

"These get you off?" he asked, kissing me fiercely.

Another nod. I didn't trust my voice.

He traced his finger down the very center of me, pressing the sodden fabric to my nether lips and my clit. I gasped. Then he pushed the panties to the side—for the point of christening them was leaving them on while we fucked—and plunged his cock inside me. My body, so wet and so ready, eased his way. When he was fully seated, the base of his cock was grinding against my clit.

"Oh," I said.

"Oh yes," he said.

Then he forgot all the dirty talk and all the play. He simply fucked me. Hard enough that we scooted together toward the head of the bed. Deep enough that I had to grip the sheets and coverlet in my clutching fingers. Hard enough that when he growled in my ear and went stiff against me, my body let loose a second rush of pleasure that was in time with his. It made the first solo orgasm seem like a distant, sweet memory.

He kissed me, pulling my bra down and delivering a lick to each perky nipple. "You like?" he asked.

"I do."

He sucked each sensitive nub and pleasure curled inside me—hot and sudden—coursing from my nipples to my gut. "I thought yellow was your color. But while I was there I saw some blue ones. Who knows? They might show up here soon."

I wiggled beneath him, excited by the prospect—and happy that he knew me so damn well.

Randy Reunion

Bethany Duggan

When I got the invitation for my ten-year college reunion, I immediately called to RSVP. I'd lost touch with most of my classmates since moving away for grad school, but I was curious to see what they were all up to, and I was overdue for a vacation.

I didn't really do much to gear up for the reunion, other than buy a new dress and get a haircut. I wouldn't have even done that much if not for my friend Karyn, who insisted I go shopping with her the weekend before the event. But, boy, am I glad I listened to her!

While I wasn't looking to impress any of my former classmates, I had always had a thing for my economics professor, Hank. He'd been fresh out of college at the time, only a few years older than his students, and he was smokin' hot. Every girl in my class had a crush on him.

Hell, I'd bet every girl in the school wanted to jump him. But he never looked twice at any of us. He was the most proper, gentlemanly guy I'd ever met—at least when I was eighteen—and had always been a welcome contrast to the immature guys on campus. I hadn't expected Hank to be at the reunion, but I'd hoped he would be, and when Karyn and I walked into the event hall, he was the first person I saw.

Hank looked older, more ruggedly handsome and not so fresh faced, but he was easy to pick out of the crowd. He still had the same piercing blue eyes and mischievous smile, and one look at him brought back all of my feelings for my college crush.

I walked around with Karyn for a while, saying hello to people we'd been in class with or had partied with years ago, but I always kept one eye on my professor, and as soon as the opportunity presented itself, I slipped away from my friend to go talk to him.

He was standing alone by the bar when I approached him, and I offered to buy him a drink before introducing myself. I told him how much I'd enjoyed his class and how even though I hadn't gone into finance, I still remembered a lot of what he'd taught me. Then, deciding I had nothing to lose, I told him about my crush. I told him how much I'd liked him, how sexy I thought he was and how aroused I was by his intelligence. I confessed that I'd fantasized about him a lot while I was in college, and that I'd always wondered what it would be like to have sex with him. He didn't say anything as I rambled on about lusting after him, so I went for broke and kissed him. That finally caused a reaction.

He kissed me for a second, and then eased me back. "Not here," he told me, and I felt my heart race as I realized what he was implying.

I finished my drink and then let him lead me out of the party and across the lawn to the library. Just past the main doors, and before the library entrance, was the freshman counseling center. It had closed during my sophomore year, and even after more than a decade, the university still hadn't found a use for the space—though my professor and I clearly had.

The counseling center was still set up like it had been all those years ago, with desks and chairs scattered around the room. It was perfect for living out my college sex fantasy.

I kissed Hank again, harder this time, and walked backward, pulling him toward the nearest desk. As soon as my thighs bumped against it, he reacted, lifting me up and setting me on the wooden surface. He pushed himself between my spread thighs and started to grind against me as we kissed, his hard cock rubbing my aching sex, with nothing between us but his slacks and my panties. It was like every fantasy I'd ever had when I was eighteen, only better, because this was real.

When I needed to breathe, I pushed him back, and while I inhaled deeply, I reached for the hem of my dress and wiggled around to free it from beneath myself and pull it over my head. Then I was sitting in front of him in only my panties (the dress hadn't gone well with any of my bras, so I went without), and the way he looked at me made me melt. I had dreamed about him ogling me that way years earlier, imagined what it would be like to have his eyes—and more—wandering over my naked body, and having it finally happen made me wetter than wet.

Hank looked me up and down for a full minute, the sexual tension between us growing, then he leaned in to kiss me while he fondled my tits. He grabbed my breasts roughly and squeezed, and the force of his touch and his kiss made me moan. His hands explored my body as we made out, our tongues battling for control. He tickled my ribs and stroked my back, then moved his hands up until his fingers were tangled in my hair and pulling me closer to him. The entire time, I felt his hard cock pressing against me through his slacks, and the sensation made me want him so much more.

I started to rub myself against him, and he quickly got the hint. He unzipped his pants and freed his dick, then pushed my panty crotch aside, baring my pussy. He looked me in the eye as he guided his cock to my entrance, and when I nodded my consent, he slammed himself inside me in one quick stroke. I yelped as his hips bumped mine; the motion was sudden, but it felt so good that my cry soon turned into a happy moan that he muffled with another deep kiss.

When he started to buck his hips, I held on and rocked with him, but as his movements became more rapid, I leaned back on my elbows and surrendered to his deep, pleasurable thrusts.

Hank was really giving it to me, fucking me harder and faster than I could remember ever being fucked, but I loved every second of it. At eighteen, I wouldn't have known what to do with that kind of frantic passion, but at thirty-two, I could take all he could give and more.

As quickly as our coupling had started, though, it ended. He'd been pounding into me so furiously that I hadn't expected either of us to last long, but we both reached orgasm much more swiftly than I'd anticipated. I came first, the fastest I'd ever climaxed, and I cried out in ecstasy as I felt my orgasm overtake me. Hank didn't stop fucking me, though, and in another thirty seconds, he was shooting off deep inside me.

When he pulled out of me a minute later, he tucked his dick back in his pants, zipped up and said we should get back to the festivities. After I pulled on my dress and straightened my hair, we exchanged phone numbers. I told him I still have some unrealized fantasies that I needed to fulfill, and he promised to help me make them all come true.

Big Spender

Rita Winchester

I crave spankings as much as Dominic craves giving them. But we've often restricted our own pleasure by only giving in to those desires with a damn good reason. However, I'll admit, I've been known to give Dominic reasons.

We'd agreed on no more spending while we got our bills in order and paid off some credit cards. I was fine with the plan and had my spending under control—until I went to a big sale on my lunch break with a friend.

There was a spectacular red sundress on sale for hardly anything at all. They were practically giving it to me at 75 percent off. There was one left, and it happened to be in my size. I bought it.

I knew what I was doing when I stopped in the restroom after work and changed from what I was wearing into the new red dress. My pussy grew wetter and wetter the closer I got to home. By the time I pulled into the driveway behind Dominic's truck, my hands were shaking. I wiggled in my seat for a moment, flexing my pussy muscles and driving my excitement higher.

Unlike a lot of men I know, Dom tends to notice things like new clothes, new haircuts, manicures and more. He's very observant and aware of me. I knew for a fact he'd notice the dress.

I swept into the house, a flurry of windblown hair, bags and nerves.

"There's my beauty." He wasn't looking at me. He was reading a piece of mail with a look of concentration on his face.

I laughed. Maybe a bit too high or a bit too wild. Because the sound I made caused him to glance up at me. I pressed my knees together to try and stabilize myself some.

"What do we have here?"

"What?" I asked. My voice was barely a whisper, and it was shivery. My voice gave me away—I knew what he was talking about.

He took a step forward, and my cunt tightened, arousal thumping through me. "The dress," he said, his voice slightly more gruff.

This time, a rush of honey escaped my pussy, and I felt as if I'd come were he to even lay a single finger on me. He grasped my arm, and I whimpered, my pulse slamming in my neck and my pussy.

"It was on sale," I said, as if that explained everything.

His lips narrowed into a thin line, and I squirmed to keep my excitement at bay. It didn't work. The motion only made matters worse.

"That's no excuse. We agreed."

"We agreed," I echoed stupidly.

"You'll need to be taught a lesson."

"A lesson," I whispered trancelike.

He released my arm and slowly slipped the dress up over my hips until it was bunched at my waist. "Take them off," Dominic said, nodding to the pale pearlescent panties I wore.

I pushed my undies down as I studied his big, strong hand gathering my pretty red dress at my waist.

"I thought you'd behave," he said conversationally. Then he slipped a hand between my thighs and brought the hard edge of his hand against my thrumming clit. I made a small noise, and he quickly shifted his hand to slide a finger into my cunt to test my wetness.

"What's worse," he said after my gasp died off, "is how much you're enjoying breaking your promise."

He let the dress drop and pointed toward the dining room with the finger slick with my juices. "Go put your hands on your dinner spot. On top of your placemat, please. Ass out. I'll be right there—to make sure you don't forget for a second time the promise you made."

I went and did as instructed. After moving aside the chair, I put my hands on the placemat at my dinner spot. I pushed my ass out and chewed my lower lip. He made me wait long enough that a fine sweat broke out on my upper lip. If I moved my legs, the slightest brush of air stroked my clitoris and made me feel like I might lose my mind.

"Stand still," he said softly from the doorway.

I froze.

Dominic came into the room, flicked my dress up with a practiced hand and began spanking me without a word, alternating strokes—right, left, right, left until my bottom thrummed with heat and blazed with pain. I found that I'd scooched myself forward and was grinding myself against the very edge of the table, trying desperately to get off.

Dom's hand stilled and moved away. "Knock it off."

Again, I froze. I was panting; I could hear my own ragged breath.

His finger drove into me from behind, and my pussy made a slick, wet sound when he entered me. I gasped, moving back to encourage him to drive his finger deeper. He added a second, flexed them once, withdrew, and then spread my own juices over my tingling clit before quickly pulling his hand away.

"Dom, please..." I was panting even louder now.

"I should punish you for real by leaving you here like this." His hand slid along the tenderness of my asscheeks. He'd spanked me for a minute, but it had been hard and no-nonsense and had caused my backside to feel as if it had been set aflame.

"Please, Dom..." I shook my head.

He began again, each strike rocketing through me, jarring my belly and making my face grow hot with arousal and helplessness. He only managed about ten more swats before he cursed and stopped. I heard his belt buckle, the urgency of his hand on his zipper.

The warm slide of his cock against my asscrack startled me, and then he was levering me forward so my body was spread over the table and my hips were trapped in his big hands. He drove into me from behind, cursing again upon entry.

My cunt was as needy as I felt inside. I intentionally tightened my internal muscles around him as he pressed his fingertips to my humming flesh. I imagined the white fingerprints that would be tattooed on the blushing skin, and I came without preamble—a jarring, surging warmth and spasm that rippled through me and left me boneless.

He grunted once, pleased, and then wiggled a moist finger into my ass. I relaxed to allow him entry. My body was invaded in two places and humming with heat and pleasure. When he thrust hard and then cried out gruffly with his own release, I came again with my breasts mashed flat to the cool wood of the tabletop.

We stayed locked together for a moment, and then Dominic stood and withdrew. He patted my ass gently, but the resulting sting caused me to sigh. I'd be aware of my punishment for hours, probably even into tomorrow. And I'd relish it.

He pulled my dress down and kissed the back of my neck where I was damp from our exertion. "By the way," he said with a chuckle. "Love the dress."

"It really was on sale," I said breathlessly.

He winked at me. "Worth every penny."

Hot Head

JAMES SATURNE

I was making a habit of coming home grumpy when my wife hit her breaking point. I came in on a particularly hot day to a very cool house, and I snapped at her. "What the hell, it's like a refrigerator in here. I know it's hot but, Jesus, Janet…"

She looked up from where she was standing over the hot stove cooking dinner. Her mouth was rigid with sudden anger.

She turned to me, put her hands on her hips and said, "Enough."

I opened my mouth, but then closed it. She'd surprised me. I'll admit it.

"Sit," she said, pointing to a chair with a wooden spoon. Her face was flushed from the steam of whatever was bubbling on the stove.

I don't know what possessed me, but without a single word, I dropped my ass in the seat and shut up.

She swished around the room in her long floral skirt and a sleeveless top that somehow made her look authoritarian.

"What's wrong with you?" she asked almost under her breath. And then she began taking my suit jacket off. I let her.

"I'm...tired," I said weakly, knowing deep down it was a piss-poor excuse for my behavior.

Janet grunted, not impressed. She took off my cufflinks, set them on the table and then rolled up my cuffs. I watched her, mesmerized but utterly unsure of what she was doing.

"Put them out," she barked, nodding toward my hands. Her voice startled me so much that I obeyed. My wife is about a foot shorter than me, petite, curvy and usually very soft-spoken.

I put my wrists out, and to my great surprise, she pulled a nylon scarf from the pocket of her skirt. She wrapped the scarf around my wrists and knotted it tightly, but not tight enough to restrict blood.

My mouth popped open but then closed. Then I repeated my fish impression again. I noticed, ironically, that my dick was hard. Not just hard. It was a rock in my pants—eager and utterly ready for action.

"I'm in no mood for your shit," she said, looking down at me. "I've had a long day, too. And then I come home, turn on the lovely air-conditioning, and proceed to cook you dinner when I'd have been happy with a cheese plate, and then you arrive barking at me?" Her lovely blue eyes narrowed in annoyance.

"I...I...um, I'm sorry," I finished weakly.

And I was. I was sorry. But I was also as horny as hell.

She studied me and cocked her head so her long, dark hair fell over her shoulder. "Fine. Prove it. Down on your knees."

"My what?" I yelped. But I noticed that my cock went from just hard to hard and desperate. My erection twitched in my pants, and before I could stifle my voice, I moaned.

She leaned in and said, "Can't you hear?"

"I...I..." There I was stammering again, and so I simply shut my mouth and tilted myself forward so that I dropped somewhat painfully to my knees. The hardwood floor was unforgiving. So was Janet because she didn't help me.

She smiled at me and then closed the space between us, her bare feet silent as she moved. She hiked up her long, gypsy skirt, and I saw that she was bare underneath. That did new and interesting things to my cock. I was leaning forward, making a rather embarrassing noise before she even uttered the sentence.

"Prove you're sorry. Eat me. Make me come."

By the time she got to the final word, I had already pressed my lips to her pussy. I nudged my tongue between her wet folds, tasted her musky loveliness. I only wished my hands were free so I could push my fingers inside her wet, velvety cunt.

The cold air-conditioning blew down on me and kept me from being miserable in what remained of my suit. The irony wasn't lost on me. To show my gratitude for the cool air, I ran the rigid tip of my tongue over her clit in perfect circles. My wrists thumped with my trapped pulse. I was sweating because I'd never been bound. I was also humping the air like a dog in heat.

"Pay attention to what you're doing," she reprimanded, threading her delicate fingers through my sweat-damp hair. She pushed her hips forward, grinding her wetness against my mouth. I shoved my tongue into her cunt, tasting how salty-sweet and hot she was there. I wanted to bury my cock inside her. I wanted to take her from behind. I wanted her to take me, riding me like a beast.

But all I could do was stay on my knees, at her mercy, and make her come.

I ate her like I never had before, my tongue darting and tasting, licking and teasing. I sucked hard, drawing on her pussy so that she whimpered. Then I released my pressure and focused my attention on her erect clit. I nipped it lightly with my teeth before teasing it with soothing strokes of my tongue. A trickle of sweat rolled down my back, and I rubbed my bound hands against my hard prick. I was so aroused I felt like I might burst.

"Jesus," she whispered, keeping my mouth and attention stable with a hand on the back of my head.

She ground against me as I lapped up her juices. She came with an uttered curse and a rush of fluids that I diligently and eagerly drank down.

She dropped to her knees, pushed me onto my back and undid my zipper. There was no time to actually take my pants off—or even remove my belt. She lifted my bound hands above my head and tilted the chair back long enough to put a leg between my bound arms. Then she set the chair back on the floor, and my wrists were ceremonially anchored by that single leg.

I found it unbelievably arousing. When she touched my cock to take it out, I moaned like I was dying.

"Don't you dare come until you give me one more," she said with eyes wild. "We're still not square."

I nodded like a madman. "Yes, yes..." I chanted.

She climbed on me, and I imagined her slick pussy leaving

marks on my dress pants. I almost came, but I managed not to—not yet.

She rode me feverishly, her hair in her eyes and her hands clutching my shoulders. I gritted my teeth, trying to rein in my pleasure. I felt like the smallest deviation in friction would make me come.

And then she began to writhe rhythmically, and I whimpered.

Janet chuckled and moved faster. She watched my face. When I shuddered and said, "Please!" she nodded, rocked her hips and came.

I lost my control then, fucking her from beneath, my hips bucking crazily. She drove down each time to meet me. The chair screeched on the hardwood from the motion of my wrists pulling at it crazily. I thrust up once more, and she leaned down and bit my nipple.

I came with a loud cry, almost knocking the chair over.

When my breathing stabilized, I looked up at her and licked my lips. "So what's for dinner?"

"Chicken cacciatore. You still pissed about the AC?"

I smiled. "Actually, it feels nice in here."

"I thought so," she said.

Dirty Delights

ALICE MUELLER

The noises emanating from the upstairs apartment were the type usually reserved for make-up sex. There were squeals, moans, sighs, catcalls, purrs, growls, hoarse whispers, and—due to an obsolete heating unit—I could hear every luscious sound.

Usually, I wouldn't have been bothered. I am all for sex. My sex. Other people's sex. I'm a fan. But I had an early morning meeting, and there was no way I could get to sleep with that racket. For the first part of the evening, I lay in bed and tried to visualize Darryl and his girlfriend in all sorts of exotic positions. What was funny is that I couldn't hear a girl's voice. Darryl definitely seemed to be taking the mic tonight.

After what I had assured myself was the last climax of the

evening—and what turned out not to be—I stomped up the stairs in my nightgown and knocked on the door.

It took a moment for my neighbor to hear me. That's because the groans had continued. I pounded. I hammered. Finally, the door opened and there stood a disheveled and quite sheepish-looking Darryl. His blond curls were matted. His blue eyes glowed.

"Oh gosh, Alice," he said, his cheeks blazing. "Did we wake you?"

"Wake me?" I repeated, dumbstruck. "Did you wake me? How could I ever have gotten to sleep? What are you doing to her?"

"Her," Darryl murmured. He sounded confused.

That's when I saw Jack. The third neighbor in our old-fashioned triplex was standing in the arched doorway wearing a pair of very rumpled black satin boxer shorts. Now I was the one to turn pink. I'd thought Darryl was straight. I'd known his ex-girlfriend—and had assumed that their on-again, off-again romance was back on once more. Meanwhile, Jack had struck me as bi; I'd seen him sometimes with men and sometimes women. I hadn't known there was anything going on between these two hunks.

"Really sorry," Jack said, ducking his head at me. "I guess we were a little noisy."

"A little," I repeated softly, but this time I was the one to sound sheepish. I have to say, all I could think about was black-haired Jack pinning blond, buff Darryl to the bed. Was one more of a top than the other? Who had been making those animalistic noises?

Darryl pulled me inside and sat me on the sofa. "Let me get you a drink to make up for the inconvenience," he said, and he disappeared into the kitchen while Jack sat across from me and kicked his bare feet up on the coffee table.

My heart was racing. I wanted in. That's what I wanted to say. *Let me in. I want to climb between you. Behind you. Show me what you were doing.* Fuck my early-morning meeting. I wanted to be spread out between them. I wanted to be the filling in a Jack-and-Darryl sandwich.

Darryl returned with a bottle of tequila and three glasses. He poured us each a golden shot while Jack continued to eye me in a way that made me feel seriously overdressed, even in only the summer-weight nightie I had on.

"So you guys are a couple..." I said, after downing my shot.

Jack smiled as Darryl said, "A couple of horny guys."

"What do you mean?"

"We went out tonight," Jack said. "Two neighbors seeing a movie. But the movie we chose was sort of sexual."

"What did you expect from a triple-X theater?" Darryl chided.

"And when we got back here..."

"Well, I was curious," Darryl said.

"I'm curious," I interrupted. There was a silence while both boys looked at me. "I mean, how did it happen? I've never heard sounds like that before."

"Well, we started to blow each other. I mean, I blew him first, and then he did me. We hadn't gotten further than that when you came pounding."

"It wasn't exactly like that," Jack said. "We were making out in the theater. We had to leave before the film ended. We were in such a rush. I guess we didn't realize how much noise we were making."

"I heard you guys. I tried to figure out who was making what sounds. I thought it was Darryl and his ex."

"No way," Darryl said, aghast. "That's over for good."

"And I hadn't heard a girl's voice."

"But you will now," Jack said, and he moved to my side and pulled my nightgown over my head and started to kiss me. I wasn't wearing any underpants, but I didn't feel exposed. I liked being naked with the two men. I closed my eyes and basked in the way Jack touched me. His hands cupped my breasts and then he started to kiss my neck. Darryl slid naturally to my other side, cradling me from behind. He scooted so that I sat down on top of him, feeling his hard cock through his drawstring pants. "I want to fuck you," I said, facing Jack but talking to Darryl. "That is, I want to fuck both of you," I said, clarifying and including Jack in the conversation so he wouldn't feel left out.

I lifted my hips and Darryl pulled his pants down. I parted my legs and sat down so that his dick was inside me. I was so wet that his rod slid in easily. I didn't know why I was so totally turned on. Maybe because of the surprise at discovering my two hunky neighbors were lovers. Or maybe because it was so obvious that they were both game to fuck me.

Then I went back to kissing Jack. Darryl put his hands on my waist and began to raise and lower me on his rock-hard cock. Jack stood and kicked off his boxers. Before he could sit again, I reached for him and positioned him in front of me. I started to blow him while Darryl fucked me. I felt overwhelmed by the pleasure of being between the two men. Plus, I remembered the noises I'd heard before, and I decided I was going to make my own erotic sounds.

With my lips wrapped around Jack's cock, I started to hum. He groaned in return, and now that all three of us were in the apartment together, he seemed to realize that he could continue to be loud.

As loud as he wanted to be. I felt myself right on the cusp of an orgasm when Darryl reached around and stroked my clit, effectively spiraling me into the sweetest climax I've ever felt. My whole body was trembling all over as Darryl pulled me off him and spun me around. Jack seemed to understand the new plan, because he got behind me and slid his cock into my slippery-wet pussy while I began to lick my juices off Darryl's slick dick.

I heard the moans that the men were making—the same type of sounds I'd eavesdropped upon earlier—and that made my heart beat faster. I was part of the mix rather than being on the outside. I was the one joining the two of them. This thought brought me to my second climax of the evening. My pussy milked Jack's cock and my mouth worked Darryl's. I had it in my head that I wanted to make the men come at the same time. I didn't speak the concept out loud—I would have had to take my mouth off Darryl's dick, and I didn't want to do that. But I hoped my neighbors would understand my X-rated mission as I began to bob faster and tighten my pussy muscles.

Jack was the one to say, "I'm coming." The way he said it, his voice so husky and raw, made me climax again. I swallowed hard as I came, and that set Darryl off, and he filled my mouth with his seed.

We moved back onto the couch afterward, overlapping, red cheeked and out of breath from the exertion of our unexpected union.

"I'm going to want to do that again," I said, as Jack bent and began to kiss my nipples.

"Oh yes," Darryl agreed enthusiastically. "But this time, I get to be in the middle."

Dripping Wet

HANNAH PERKINS

I was running on the treadmill when I saw Brittany come out of the locker room. I watched her make her way across the gym in the large mirror that ran along the wall, and I noticed that the guy on the treadmill two down from mine was doing the same thing. As she continued her approach, I looked down the line of joggers and then glanced up in the mirror to check out the people on the bikes and ellipticals behind me. Almost every man in the room was watching my girlfriend as she strutted down the aisle between the machines in her tight leggings and sports bra. Her workout attire left little to the imagination, and the way she walked made it clear that she was open to being ogled.

One of the guys catcalled her as she went past, and Brittany turned and blew him a kiss. But she wasn't interested in him—or any of the other guys. Nope, the hot aerobics instructor who had the attention of all the men was only interested in one gym rat—me. She winked at me in the mirror as she strolled by on her way to teach her class, and I smiled back before hitting the button on the machine a few times and picking up my pace.

Brittany and I had made a bet a few days earlier. Only a couple of months into our relationship, we'd been fucking like bunnies, getting it on anywhere and anytime we could. As girls, it was easy enough. We could disappear into the bathroom together at nightclubs and restaurants without anyone thinking twice, and fucking in department-store dressing rooms was a simple thrill. Our friends, however, were getting tired of walking in on us. So we'd decided to see how long we could go without sex. The first one to cave and make a move on the other would lose. So far, we'd gone three days, but it wasn't easy. To keep the sexual tension at bay, I'd taken to working out nonstop. I'd thought for sure that would help, but with Brittany constantly strutting around the gym where we both worked in her barely there workout clothes, I had a feeling I'd be throwing in the towel before the end of the week.

Wednesday was always the longest day of the week for both of us. My girlfriend had six classes to teach, and I was responsible for running orientation sessions for new members, so we basically spent the whole day in the gym. Normally, that wasn't a problem, but being in such close proximity while we were getting hot and sweaty was not going to make our bet any easier for me to win. By noon, I'd already run more than ten miles, and I still had hours to go before my shift ended. The fact that Brittany was taking every opportunity to waltz past me in her skimpy outfit didn't help matters, either. I swear she walked an extra half-dozen miles that day just to drive me crazy.

My last orientation session ended at seven o'clock, and I was grateful for the fact that Brittany had a spin class until eight, giving me an hour to do paperwork and maybe not think about my incredibly sexy girlfriend. I got all the new clients' info entered in our database and wiped down all the equipment so the late-night manager wouldn't have as much work. Then I disappeared into the employees-only locker room to shower.

As the hot water streamed down on me, I couldn't help thinking about my girlfriend's ass, rising up and down on the spinning bike only a few yards away on the gym floor. Without thinking about it, I reached down between my legs and started rubbing my pussy. My juices were dripping freely out of me, and I swiped them up with a finger before thrusting my digit into my slit. In the time that Brittany and I had been together, we hadn't gone more than twenty-four hours without at least a little friendly groping, so three days felt like an eternity.

I got so caught up in my spur-of-the-moment masturbation session that I didn't hear the key in the door or the squeak of the hinges as someone else entered the locker room. I didn't hear the slap of bare feet on the tiled floor or the whoosh of the shower curtain being pulled back. It wasn't until I felt the water go suddenly cold that my attention returned from my daydream to reality.

Brittany had snuck up on me and caught me, and she had decided that I needed a cold shower. Now I was being pelted by icy water as my girlfriend laughed. But she wasn't laughing for long. When I turned to give her hell, she found herself face-to-face with my naked, wet tits—and I found myself looking at my equally nude girlfriend. At almost the same time, we leaned in and started to kiss. And we weren't sharing the stupid little pecks we'd taken to since we started our bet; we were full-on making out.

When our hands started to explore each other's curves, Brittany stepped into the shower with me. Now closer than we'd allowed ourselves to be in seventy-two hours, we pressed our bodies right up against each other and stroked every inch of skin we could reach. Our mouths soon followed suit, and we began trailing kisses all over each other's wet flesh. We were a mess of lips and limbs as we each tried to get what we wanted and bumped and jostled each other in the process. We were so desperate for each other that we didn't even think to turn on the hot water again; our bodies were hot enough even under the cool spray.

Eventually, we realized that we needed to move in a more synchronized fashion, and I let Brittany push me up against the wall, where we ground our pussies together and feasted on each other's breasts. When the frantic humping wasn't enough to sate us, I reached down and began caressing my girlfriend's pussy. I slipped two fingers inside her and stroked her, reaching for her G-spot, and she released my tit to gasp out loud. She copied me a moment later, pushing two of her digits between my thighs and pumping them furiously in and out of my cunt.

Our fingers moved frantically as we tried to bring each other to climax, and when we leaned in to kiss again, our teeth clicked together as our passion took on a new urgency. Brittany's free hand continued to massage my right breast as we kissed and finger-fucked each other, and mine went to her ass, roughly kneading her firm cheeks.

I was so hungry for her—and so desperate to come—my pussy began spasming in no time, and I felt my whole body quake as my orgasm took over. I kissed Brittany even harder as I came, needing to silence the screams of ecstasy that were threatening to escape my lips. A few moments later, she climaxed, too, shivering in my arms.

We continued writhing against each other as we came down from our orgasmic highs, and we heard someone behind us cursing. I turned my head in time to catch our friend and coworker, Janet, walking away. We were busted—again.

Brittany and I disagreed on who caved first that day, but we had to agree that even though one of us had technically lost the bet, we both felt like winners.

That Kind of Girl

JENNIFER PETERS

I crawled down the bed and watched as Ryan's cock twitched. I could hear him breathing heavily, but I couldn't drag my eyes away from his engorged dick to see if I'd successfully wiped the look of shock off his face.

Technically, we'd been on our first date earlier that night, but considering we'd been flirting with each other for the past three years, it was hard for me to accept that all our late-night video-game sessions and after-work happy hours didn't count as dates. Still, we'd never done more than share quick, friendly kisses on New Year's Eve, so that part of the date was new. And neither of us had planned on ending up in bed together at the end of the night.

It had been my decision. When Ryan asked what we should

do after dinner, I suggested we go back to his place. I don't know what came over me, but after all those years of playing around and not quite dating, I suddenly found myself wanting my friend in a way I never had before. He'd put up a fight. He thought we should go for a walk on the beach, or maybe see a movie. He said he wanted to "do things right" with me, which meant no sex on the first date because, as he kept pointing out, I wasn't "that kind of girl." It took a little convincing to get him to understand that I wanted him, and I didn't care how many dates we hadn't been on. He quickly came around to seeing things my way.

He'd been so ecstatic, in fact, that he'd made it his mission to bring me to orgasm right away. After he'd gotten me naked and in his bed, he went down on me. I'd been with plenty of guys before Ryan, but only a couple had ever eaten my pussy, and none of them had done it with the same level of enthusiasm. He licked me gently at first, and then more firmly. I'd never felt anything as good as his tongue lapping up my juices from my pussy lips. When he moved his mouth up to suck on my clit, I came instantly. It felt so amazing, but he didn't stop there.

I thought for sure he'd move on to another activity once I'd reached orgasm, but Ryan looked up at me, grinning, and went right back to licking and sucking my sensitive bud. While his mouth was busy with my clit, he brought a hand between my legs and started stroking my pussy. When he slipped one of his thick fingers inside me, I moaned and fisted his sheets. I expected him to be good in bed—he'd had a reputation as a ladies' man for as long as I'd known him—but oh my god! I never imagined anyone could bring me the kind of pleasure that Ryan was giving me.

He started thrusting his finger in and out of me rapidly, and

I bucked my hips against his hand, forcing his digit even deeper. His attention never wavered from my pussy, and when I came a second time, he stayed between my thighs until he'd licked me clean.

When he came back up to lie next to me, I leaned over to kiss him and tasted myself on his lips. It was the most erotic experience, and I quickly peppered kisses all over his face, planting my lips everywhere I saw my juices shining on his skin.

We shared one more deep lip-lock, and then he got up to get us a couple of bottles of water. We finished our drinks quickly, and then I told him I wanted to return the favor. He started in again about how I didn't have to do anything I didn't want to and how I wasn't "that kind of girl," but I assured him that I *did* want to. I *was* that kind of girl. He looked surprised, but he didn't say anything more.

I pushed Ryan onto his back and kissed a trail down his body, stopping first at his nipples, which I sucked gently, and then at his navel, which I traced several times with the tip of my tongue. When I moved lower, I trailed my fingers along the soft path of blond hairs that led from his stomach to his cock, and then I sucked the tip of him into my mouth. I heard Ryan gasp loudly as my lips wrapped around his dick, and I smiled around his shaft, happy that I was able to elicit such a reaction.

Ryan's cock was thicker and longer than I'd envisioned, so I couldn't deep-throat him, although I tried. It didn't seem to bother him, though. When I wrapped a hand around his erection, keeping my mouth at the tip, he moaned loudly again, letting me know I was doing a good job.

I ran my hand up and down his length, going from the base right up to my lips and then back down. Sometimes I'd twist my hand a bit at the top or bottom, or I'd tighten my grip and squeeze, wanting to keep him on edge. I did that over and over, maybe a dozen times, and then I pulled my mouth off his dick and ducked my head down to suck one of his balls between my lips. I continued to stroke his shaft as I swirled my tongue around first one ball and then the other, and Ryan grunted.

I could tell he was getting close when he started thrusting his hips, so I moved my mouth from his balls back to his cockhead. I sucked him into my mouth again and let him buck upward so he was fucking my face. When he realized what I was doing, he slowed his thrusts as much as he could, being careful not to go too deep.

When he was ready to climax, he tried to pull me away from his cock. He pushed on my shoulders and told me to let go, but I continued sucking him. Finally, he yelled, "God, I'm about to come! You have to stop!" but I didn't. I pulled my mouth back enough to mumble, "I want this," and then sucked him back down. When he shot his load a moment later, I swallowed as much of his cream as I could before pulling away and letting him spew the rest on my tits.

Ryan pulled me up and wrapped his arms around me, kissing me passionately and mashing our chests together—not caring that he was getting come all over himself. "God, you're amazing!" he said.

By the time we'd caught our breath, Ryan's cock was half hard again. I stroked him, pleasantly surprised by his speedy recovery, and had his dick standing at attention in only a few seconds. He reached over to his nightstand to get a condom out of the drawer, ripped it open and rolled it onto his shaft. Then he positioned himself on top of me, his hard-on brushing against my wet center. He pushed inside me in one smooth stroke, and then to my intense delight, he fucked me.

I had three orgasms that night with Ryan—two more than I'd ever had with anyone else. By the time we went on our third official date, we were experts in getting each other off. But that doesn't stop me from occasionally reminding my boyfriend that, if it had been up to him, he'd never have discovered exactly what kind of girl I really am.

Corrective Measures

Sam Morris

"You weren't kidding when you said we received a major shipment."

"This morning, you couldn't even take a step forward," Megan told me, standing at my side and shaking her head in sympathy.

"I believe you," I said, making my way through the boxes. The huge cartons were everywhere. As I walked around the room, I kept shaking my head in disbelief. We'd never been swamped with a shipment like this before. I couldn't see my desk. Christ, I couldn't even see my coworker. I'd left her behind me as I made my way through the maze.

"What the fuck?" I asked nobody in particular.

"They got the numbers wrong," Megan said from somewhere deep in box city.

"*Really* wrong."

"Yeah, like ten times off." She found me in what I supposed was the center of the room.

"How could you let this happen?"

"The bill of lading was correct," she said. "I double-checked. Only when I called the home office did I realize the error."

"You didn't notice when you couldn't see the windows anymore?"

"I thought maybe it was for a new promotion."

I sighed. Nobody likes Mondays anyway, right? And now I had more inventory than I'd ever seen before.

"They have to come take it back," I said, thinking that whatever I'd planned to get done that day would have to wait.

"Not until tonight."

"We're supposed to work like this?"

She shrugged.

"Is anyone else here?"

"We're the only ones."

The way she said the words made me pause. "Really?"

"Yup. Really." Then she said something that made my stiffening cock twitch in my khakis. "I'm sorry I messed up, Sam."

"How sorry?" I asked as my cock went to full mast.

"So very sorry." She was undressing as she spoke. I knew that this was a dangerous game, but I didn't have the heart to stop it. Not when Megan bent over the nearest box and looked at me over her shoulder. "I know you'll need to punish me for being so careless."

I started to pull the belt from the loops of my pants. I couldn't wait to tear open my slacks and get inside her. But we'd played this scenario before. The redder Megan's bottom, the harder she comes.

"Ten with the belt seems about right," I told her. "What do you think?"

She arched her back in answer, spreading her legs and getting herself situated. I came closer and touched her bare pussy with my fingertips. She was already drenched.

"You were fantasizing about what would happen to you, weren't you, while you watched them deliver all these boxes?"

"Yup," she admitted.

"And did you play with yourself while you imagined my reaction?" I kept probing her pussy while I spoke. Megan was sighing and shivering. I could imagine that the box below her was going to have a wet spot by the time we were through.

"I waited until the truck drove away. Then I went to the restroom and made myself come. I knew you'd see red when you came in today."

"Oh, I'm going to see red all right," I said, and I landed the first blow on her naked asscheeks. She jumped and swore under her breath, then got herself right back into position. That's one of my favorite things about punishing Megan. She can't hide how much she craves the spark of pain and the instantaneous wave of pleasure that follows it.

I cracked the belt against her sweet ass a second time, and she hissed under her breath. I had to stop then to feel her pussy once more. "You're so fucking wet," I told her, as I made her lick her juices off my fingertips. "I don't think you consider this punishment at all."

She had no answer to that. I striped her again and again. We were at four, only four, but I had to be inside her. I picked her off the first box and pushed her over a taller one, this container at the perfect height for me. "I'm not done spanking you," I told her, "but I've got to fuck you first." I undid my slacks and pulled out my dick, not bothering to undress all the way. Megan was naked enough for both of us. I spread her thighs with my hands, and I slid the head of my cock inside her.

"Oh sweet Jesus," Megan moaned. She was almost coming from the first touch. I didn't tell her not to; I'm not that cruel. I rocked in and out of her, and I brought one hand between the box and her pussy to give her a few fingers to press against. She lined her clit up with my knuckles and ground her hips against my hand. I kept fucking her while she got herself off, and then I pulled out and gripped my belt once more.

"You didn't come," she said, her voice hoarse.

"No, not yet. I'm going to shoot all over your red-hot bottom and rub my come into your skin," I told her. She gazed at me over her shoulder, and I saw that my words were turning her on even more. "You like that," I said. "Don't you? You like to feel that sticky come on your hot asscheeks?"

"Yes, Sir," she said, and she writhed a little to let me know she was ready.

"Touch yourself while I punish you," I instructed, and she immediately got her greedy little hand between her legs and started tickling her clit while I lined up the next few blows. I was counting them off in my head. I knew Megan must be, as well. For the last one, I made her hold open her asscheeks and I tapped the belt lip against her asshole. Her body bucked, and I rewarded her by dropping to my knees and pressing my lips to her pucker.

"Oh god," she whimpered. "Tongue me, Sir. Tongue me!"

I rimmed her good, and we both knew what that meant. Megan was wet enough that I was able to scoop up her juices on my fingers and jack my cock with her personal lubrication. I pulled her asscheeks open wide and introduced her to the head of my cock. She stilled totally, her fingers stopped working over her clit, and even her breath seemed to halt in her chest. Then I pushed forward and she relaxed, accepting me. Spanking Megan always makes me want to take her ass. I don't know what it is about seeing those striped cheeks that ramps up my craving for anal. But we both know this is how any spanking event will always end.

I powered my cock in and out of her back channel, and she whinnied and tossed her hair as she resumed toggling her clit.

When I told her to come, she did, and I imagined I saw flickers of gold dancing in the air around her, a halo of pleasure that was visible in its intensity. I waited her out, and then I plunged once more, withdrew, and jerked my cock so that I sprayed my white cream all over her asscheeks, exactly as I'd promised I would.

We basked in a moment of total silence—then we slowly caught our breath. Surrounded by the sea of cardboard boxes, we'd created our own little sliver of paradise, but we knew we couldn't stay like this all day. I went to the restroom to clean myself up, and when I came back, Megan was dressed once more. She said, "The truck will be here by five to pick up the overage. They just called. Hopefully, those two boxes will have dried by then."

I looked and saw that she had indeed left wet spots on both of the cartons we'd played on. I didn't have a problem with that. But I promised to punish her after hours for her indiscretion. Megan shot me a happy smile and wiggled her ass as she went off in search of her desk.

Sultry Sex Ed

Jenna Lui

The start of a new semester is always my favorite time of year. The campus fills up with hundreds of sexy students, and I have my pick of hookup partners. It never takes me long to line up my first few dates, but as I was scoping out potentials in the registration office, someone unexpected caught my eye.

Sitting behind the desk was the loveliest woman I had ever seen. She looked older, maybe in her forties, but thanks to her tight sleeveless top, I could clearly see her fit figure. She had her hair pulled up in a loose bun, a pencil stuck through the middle holding it in place, and she was wearing a striking pair of red-framed glasses. It was lust at first sight, and I couldn't wait for the line to move up so I could finally come face-to-face with this alluring cougar.

There were only three people ahead of me, and the cougar—whose name, I later learned, was Linda—was quick to remedy their problems and get to me. After I had her switch my morning history class for an afternoon block, I did my best to flirt with her. I chatted her up about her job and how difficult it must be, and I asked her when she worked so I'd know when to come back if I needed help again.

A few days later, I swung by the registration office right after closing, hoping to run into Linda again. I got lucky—as I approached the building, she came out the front door. I ran up to her and asked if she was leaving for the day. I acted surprised when she pointed out that it was already after five o'clock. I told her I'd been hoping to get help logging in to my account, since it seemed I'd been locked out. "I knew I should've written down my password," I told her, feigning annoyance.

She looked at me for a moment, and I pushed out my chest and stood up extra straight, making sure she got the full picture. Then she turned around and headed back toward the door, telling me to come with her. "I think I forgot to turn off my computer anyway," she said. "And this should only take a minute."

I smiled. My plan was working. After she checked my account and reset my password, she turned off her computer and walked out with me. I thanked her profusely and then asked if I could buy her a cup of coffee for staying late to help me. She said it was too late for coffee, so I suggested a drink instead. I worried for a second that she'd say no, but then she looked me over again, really checking me out, and finally agreed. "Sure," she said. "I could use a drink."

We went to the wine bar down the street—conveniently located a block away from my apartment—and had a couple of glasses of cabernet. I pulled out all the stops as we talked and flirted, making sure there was no mistaking exactly what I wanted. Linda seemed to be on the same page, and it wasn't long before I felt her high heel-clad foot running up and down my leg. When her hand came to rest on my knee and she began caressing my thigh, I knew it was time to make my move. I placed my hand on her leg and then leaned forward. When she didn't immediately back away, I moved in closer, and I didn't stop until my lips were pressed firmly against hers.

Linda kissed me back, softly at first and then with more passion. Soon her tongue was exploring my mouth, and before I knew it, I was getting wet in my jeans. When we broke apart to gasp for air, I suggested we go somewhere more private, and without a moment's hesitation, Linda agreed. We settled our tab, and then I guided Linda to my apartment.

Once inside and alone, my cougar pounced. She was on me in a flash, her hot mouth searing against mine and her hands roaming freely over my body. I like to be in charge, but I had no issue with a sexy older woman taking the lead. She had at least twenty years of experience on me, and I was eager to learn anything she could teach me.

I followed her lead, my hands tracing the same path on her body that she was creating on mine, and when she deepened our kiss, I moved my tongue in sync with hers as well. She teased me for a while, keeping me there in the living room as we kissed and caressed each other. Soon enough, her desire for more won out. During a brief pause in our lip-lock, she whispered, "Bedroom." I pulled back, grabbed her hand and led her to my room at the back of the apartment.

We had barely crossed the threshold into the bedroom when she started tugging at my clothing, undressing me. I once again followed suit, my fingers grabbing at her dress and then her lingerie, helping her shed every garment until she was completely naked. As soon as the last barriers were out of the way, Linda pushed me down onto my full-size bed and climbed on top of me.

I'd been thinking about having her naked body pressed against mine since I'd first laid eyes on her, but the reality was even better than the fantasy. Her breasts were round but soft, and when she lowered her body to mine, her tits pressed deliciously against my own. She had a fuller bush than I did, too, and as she ground against me, the downy hair tickled my skin. We hadn't even done anything yet, and already I was more turned on than I'd been in ages.

Once we were horizontal, we spent only a few moments savoring the feeling of our bodies pressing tightly together before our lip-lock resumed, and then our hands took up their explorations once more. I groped Linda's tight ass, letting my fingers knead her flesh while hers tickled my ribs and then fondled my breasts. But it still wasn't enough. Luckily, Linda and I were still on the same page, and as the first flash of frustration flitted through my mind, she began shifting around until we were in a sixty-nine. *Ahh*, I thought, *much better.*

As soon as her pussy appeared in front of my face, I pulled her hips down, impaling her cunt on my stiff tongue. She was dripping wet—I'm sure I was, too—and after tongue-fucking her for a moment, I lapped up all the flavorful juices that clung to her labia. Then I dove right back in, my lips and tongue working over her with a renewed sense of fervor. I couldn't get enough!

At the same time, Linda's mouth was moving nonstop, and her tongue was doing things to me I can't begin to describe. I'd never felt so much pleasure, not all at once, and I marveled at what an incredible lover she seemed to be. My thoughts didn't last long, though—it was impossible to think with her tongue bringing me to new heights. The ecstasy I was experiencing was so far beyond anything I'd ever dreamed of that it took every ounce of willpower I had to keep my own tongue working between her thighs.

I was on the verge of an orgasm in no time, and I gave myself over to the sensations. When Linda sucked my clit between her full lips, I came. I groaned loudly, and then I let go. My entire body tingled with the sense of release.

I lay there beneath her for several seconds, relishing the orgasmic high she'd brought me to, but once the fog cleared, I returned my attention to Linda's pussy. It was my turn to get her off.

As my tongue pumped between her pussy lips, I grabbed her ass again, softly massaging her flesh until my fingertips reached her crack. I spread her cheeks gently, and then I began tracing her crimped backdoor with a spit-slickened finger. I heard her moan happily, and when I felt her relax a little more against me, I pushed my digit past the tight muscle and into her rear entrance. My tongue never stopped working her pussy as my finger slowly probed her ass, and from the way she was writhing against me, I knew she was getting close. I moved my tongue to her clit, licking firmly, and then started wiggling my finger inside her backdoor. With a moan, she climaxed.

I sucked down every drop of sweet juice that poured into my mouth, and when there was no more, I licked Linda's pussy clean. Then I came up for air.

Linda had to get going after that, but she let me know that she hoped we'd "run into each other" again soon—and I'm certain that we will.

Horny Homecoming

Peter McLoughlin

When I can manage it, I come home a day or two earlier than promised from my out-of-town business trips. I text my wife, Jessie, before I board the plane, and she makes sure I have a good homecoming.

We do this once or twice a year, and we look forward to our special time as much as birthdays and Christmas. Making this sort of playtime a rare treat also keeps it special.

When I returned from my recent trip to Wisconsin, I pulled into the driveway and saw a red sports car parked outside that didn't belong to either of us. I knew Jessie would later tell the neighbors that our guest was a visiting relative or a long-ago frat brother of mine, but I knew who he truly was as I climbed out of the car: he was the man currently fucking my wife.

Knowing Jessie, they were probably still entangled in foreplay. She'd no doubt timed every act perfectly, so I could get home and make my grand entrance in order to view the main event. I wasn't quiet about entering our home, giving Jessie plenty of time to work up our visitor.

When I came to stand in the bedroom, there they were. He looked a bit stunned—naked as the day he was born—with my wife's leg in his hand. She was nude but for a smile, her wrists tied to the headboard with some red rope.

"Hey, baby," she cooed.

Her lover didn't say anything. He just stared at me, gauging what I might do. Would I be angry? Would I come at him? Would I do anything crazy?

I dropped my bag. "Hey," I replied. I took off my tie, nodded to him and then put my tie on the dresser. I took my time and moved slowly, as if I had all the time in the world. Because I did. As long as he didn't run, we'd be fine. As long as my wife's pussy was more important to him than his worry.

We'd only ever had one guy run, and one out of about a dozen or so isn't too terrible.

"This is Max," she said. "He's here to have fun. I told him you like to watch, baby. Now you tell him. Or I think he might leave."

I began to unbutton my shirt. I gave Max another nod and smiled. "I like to watch. You go ahead and do whatever you were about to do."

He looked dubious, but then Jessie raised her hips, effectively drawing his attention back to her naked body. She wiggled for him and whispered, "Bring that big dick back up here for me to suck."

His eyes went from her to me and then from me to her. He looked uncertain, but who can blame him. Jessie raised her hips again and whispered "Dick," and he groaned. Then he was straddling my wife, moving up her body, his cock once again as hard as a stone and aimed right for her mouth.

Who could argue with logic like Jessie wanting to suck you off?

I dropped into the chair by the foot of the bed. It was placed at the perfect angle—one Jessie and I had spent a whole Saturday perfecting—so that I could see everything from pussy-eating to cock-sucking to full-on penetration. Occasionally, I had to move a few inches to the left or right, but that was a rare occurrence.

She lifted her head up to take him deeper, and I felt the ache of lust and arousal in my balls and belly. I held my breath as she gagged—just a little—on his girth. Her eye makeup was running perfectly, giving her the effect of an ink-and-water painting. She moaned, and I had to hold my breath to keep from following suit.

Sometimes, I marvel at the fact that Jessie is mine. That she chose me. And nothing brings that home more than when some guy's fucking her right in front of me, and I know that her mind is all about making sure I get the show I want. The show I need.

Then it's all about me and her. Usually, for a few days we barely come up for air.

I refocused myself on the action, just in time to see him rear up farther and push his balls against her lips. She sucked one then the other, making sure to drag her tongue down the tender skin that separated one testicle from the other.

He growled deep in his throat, sounding like some wild thing we'd brought home. I saw him almost turn to look at me but then catch himself. He would pretend I wasn't there. The best ones always did.

He released her from her bonds and practically barked at her, "On your hands and knees."

He'd fuck her doggie-style to show his dominance. I rested my hand on my fly, feeling the pulse and thump of my erection; it seemed to radiate through my hand, though I thought that was more my imagination.

I would watch, and I would wait, and when we ushered him out, I'd fuck her. Wring orgasm after orgasm out of her, while the smell of a stranger hung in the air and she told me what they'd done together before I got home.

Max ran his cockhead from her pussy to her ass, and then back down again. He reached under her to stroke a clitoris I knew would be swollen with arousal. He must have pinched her because she practically purred and said, "Oh yeah, I like it that way."

I dragged my flattened palm along my hard-on but didn't do anything more. Just that pressure, just that friction, was all I was allowed.

He sucked on his finger and then put it in her asshole, and I found that I was holding my breath. He pulled free and then inserted his pointer and his middle fingers together. As he did that, Max slid his cock into her pussy gradually, taking his time penetrating her. I could tell by the set of his shoulders that he was aware of me but didn't want to look in my direction.

I breathed out slowly—a jittering kind of exhalation.

Max grabbed her hip with his free hand, anchoring her in place so he could drive in deep. His hips moved fast, his body smacking against hers so loudly it was almost like the sound of clapping. I watched his cock—hard and wet—sliding in and out, in and out of my wife. His fingers mimicked that same motion, driving in and out of her ass hard enough to make her toss her head back.

"Yeah, baby. Like that," Jessie said.

I bit my tongue to sharpen my focus and to help me keep my hands off my dick. I dragged my hand along my length again, my eyes drifting shut a little as I relished the sensation.

"Goddamn it," he said. Most likely he was more turned on by me being there than he cared to admit. Fucking a man's beautiful wife *in front of* that man? How could that not be a turn-on for a macho guy like Max?

The tattoo on his left shoulder flexed with his efforts, and he hissed. He was going to come. He reached under her again, rubbing her clit harder, and she shoved herself back to take his big cock. Then her head was down and her hair was flying and she was crying out in the throes of her orgasm.

"On my ass. Come on my ass." She chanted her words as he delivered his final few strokes. With a snarl, our visitor pulled free of her cunt and shot his load all over her asscheeks and even her back hole. She'd pried her cheeks apart for him to get that money shot.

Max would carry that visual with him for a while, I was fairly certain.

I left the room and let her say her goodbyes. In the bathroom, I washed my face, brushed my teeth, and stripped off the rest of my clothes. She'd suck me off, and I'd come fast. I'd come hard. And then we'd make a point of lying there together and getting ourselves worked up for a good leisurely fuck.

"Coming, baby?" she called.

I could hardly wait. I wasn't sure what was better: the show she'd put on for me, the promise of future ones or...the sex we were about to have. All I know is I'm a very, very lucky man.

Back to Basics

PENELOPE CHEVALIER

Last week, my boyfriend, Jason, surprised me. Literally. He made me gasp when I walked in the apartment and he was suddenly there, right behind me. "Arms out in front of you, baby girl. Daddy brought you a new toy."

I shivered. It was an automatic response to the word "Daddy." I put my arms out in front of me and stood there, trying to keep my knees from buckling as he stripped me right there in the foyer and bound my wrists. When I was bare but for my heels, he put a black blindfold around my eyes, tying it tight behind my head.

"Come on, now," he said, walking me gently forward and into the kitchen. He moved and turned me until I felt the back of my hips hit the cool marble countertop, and then he was lifting me.

I bit my lip to keep from crying out. I was always to trust Daddy. Never to worry. So any sort of noise would have been bad.

He'd been watching me closely because he said, "You're such a good girl, trusting your Daddy completely."

"What did you get me?" I asked. I had to ask. I could hear him rummaging in a bag as I sat there, bare-assed and desperate on our kitchen counter.

"Something I think you'll like." And then he tsked. "Now you know you're supposed to wait for me to surprise you."

"I'm sorry," I said, but I wasn't. Not really. My pulse beat heavy with anticipation. Was it a crop? A paddle? A vibrator? A dildo?

The possibilities were limitless because Jason likes to play with me. He likes to get me wet—not wet, drenched—and then fuck me. It's his favorite pastime, and I never have an objection.

"I was in a meeting the other day where we were discussing the basics. Going back to simple things."

I made a noise, waiting. Ready. Aching.

"And I realized I missed simple things. Cheese and grapes for dinner with a bottle of wine—the way we used to. Or, you know—back before everyone walked around with a phone and a tablet all wired up to WiFi—just walking out of the house with only my keys."

Jason turned me slightly, so I was facing away from him. I was sprawled out on the marble like some sort of food offering. Then he pulled me back so I was leaning against him. Jason parted my legs slightly, and I felt the cool kiss of what I guessed was some sort of sex toy.

"Spread your legs."

I did as instructed, and he stroked my clit with the impersonal plastic device. But then he pinched my nipples, and I gasped.

"I went back to basics. I kept it simple. What we have here is a plain white, plastic vibrator."

The sound of the toy coming to life fully filled our large kitchen. The noise seemed to ricochet around the room like a confused bird in flight.

"These things were sold in the back of nearly every damn magazine not so long ago. And even in those clever women's household catalogs. Back then, they were always called 'personal massagers.' Do you remember?"

I could only nod because he was running the pulsating tip of the toy against my clitoris. Then he outlined the ridges of my pussy lips with it before pulling the toy away and running it along my shoulder, my clavicle, my arm.

"They showed women using it on their shoulders." He was laughing outright now. "And their shins. Not to mention, my personal favorite, their eyebrows."

I giggled despite my anticipation. He'd eventually tire of running that buzzing thing along my skin and run it lower, where I needed it most—I hoped.

Then he ran the vibe over the blindfold. I jumped when it slipped down to touch my face, but Jason shushed me, kissed my temple and stroked my clitoris with his fingertips. A moan broke free of me, and he slid the toy down my cheek and neck. He traced my nipple, forcing that halo of tender flesh to perk up. The buzzing plastic meandered down the center of my chest to my belly button and then my mound. Jason pressed the vibrator to my mons until the buzzing seemed to fill me from cunt to chest. The rumbling sensations echoed all through me; even my lips seemed to be absorbing the rhythmic pulses.

When I thought I'd start to cry—or maybe even scream—he pressed the vibrator to my clit and held it there. He must have thumbed the button because the speed ratcheted up from the lowest setting to the highest in an instant. I sobbed and my hips rose.

"Too much," I whispered. "Oh god—"

"Hush," he said. "Just a second. If it's still too much in a second I'll turn it—"

Another moan fell from my lips because what had been overwhelming quickly turned pleasurable. I found myself moving up to meet the toy. He kissed my neck, still holding me to him in a protective gesture.

"I want you to come," he said, letting me know this wasn't a denial game. I nodded eagerly. *That* I could do.

He swirled the tip of the wildly jumping contraption against my clit, only moving it away and along my outer lips and my slit to give my clit a break. Then he'd return to that sensitive nub and a whole new rush of sensations would overtake me.

"Spread them wider," he said and I obeyed. My legs were practically splayed on the counter, my calves hanging down and my upper body resting against him. And for a brief and fascinating flash in my mind, I imagined a whole viewing audience seated before the kitchen island I was perched on. A whole ring of watchers around us as he tortured me with pleasure.

When he held the vibrator in place with no reprieve on the horizon and said softly, "Come for me," I did. Just as if he'd said "pour the wine" or "preheat the oven" or "open the door." *Come for me* was a command I had no problem following.

"Now when I fuck you with this," he whispered before I was

even finished with my orgasm, "I want you to touch yourself. You're so pretty all spread out like this. So pretty and so filthy at the same time."

His words, oh fuck, his words did as much for me as any touch he could deliver. As any sex we could possibly have. The words he gave to me on a regular basis were as enticing as his fingers in my pussy or his mouth on my nipple.

The vibrator slid inside me with ease. I was so drenched. Jason drove it deep, and the top of the toy pounded my G-spot so that warmth spread through my arms and legs and belly. I lazily stroked my clit until it wasn't enough. I used a firmer hand, adding more pressure.

Jason angled the device a little, and I cried out. My fingers moved a bit faster, despite my bound wrists. He swirled the toy deep inside me, and I rubbed faster still. But I gave up when he pulled the vibrator almost out of me and then plunged it back in. I climaxed wildly, saying his name over and over.

I was breathless and boneless as he rearranged us, standing me up and pushing me forward, with my bound hands trapped between my hips and the island. He knocked my legs wide and yanked my hips up so I stood on tiptoe. I held my position as he drove into me, grunting. Any pretense was gone. He was all about the fucking now. All about his release.

His abandon thrilled me so much my nipples spiked hard against the marble counter.

"Perfect," he rasped. "You're fucking perfect when you come." And then he surrendered to his climax. My body offered up a small, soft orgasm in conjunction with his.

When he took the blindfold off, he turned me and waved the

plain-Jane, white vibe in my face. "What did you think about my old-school idea?"

My legs were shaky. "I loved it," I answered. My voice matched my legs.

He grinned. "Good, because I have my eye on a hank of old-fashioned hemp rope. No frills. And it has your name written all over it." He kissed me. "Sound good?"

I nodded, kissing him back. "Sounds perfect." And it did.

Making New Memories

MITCH RODGERS

When I walked into the living room and found Belinda with a man I didn't recognize, I paused.

"Honey, this is Dan. He and I went to school together back in the day."

Belinda always said "back in the day" as if she were in her sixties instead of her early twenties. I shook the man's hand and offered him a beer. He accepted. It was when I came back that I noticed he looked a bit nervous.

"Everything okay?" I asked, handing over the cold bottle.

"Fine," answered my wife. "I told Dan you'd be okay with my proposition, but you know no one ever believes us."

That was when the lightbulb went on over my head. I laughed softly. "Oh, yeah—especially the men."

She nodded. "See, Dan, I told you!" She patted his leg.

"We're down with threesomes," I said, trying to keep my tone light.

"We've done another woman for him," Belinda said, tilting her head my way. I raised my beer to Dan who still looked uncertain but no longer downright terrified.

"And we've done an extra guy for me," she said smiling. "And I'd like you to be another guy for us."

"The only rule is I don't really have any contact with you," I said. "That's not my deal. I mean dicks do accidentally touch from time to time, and no worries—that doesn't concern me. Just a heads-up that this is *us* fucking *her*. Not us fucking her and each other."

Dan nodded and swallowed hard, and then said, "That's fine. I mean, that's how I'd want it. Not that..." He shook his head, laughing. "Never mind." After two big swallows of beer, he said to Belinda, "When would you want to do it?"

"How about now?" she said, eyes lighting up like it was Christmas.

I laughed. "She has no patience. I don't know if you recall."

He nodded, almost smiling. "I'm starting to."

Belinda stood and took off her dress. It was a warm day, so one zip and she was out of her white-and-yellow shift. Beneath, she wore only a pair of pale-blue panties.

I made a noise in my chest that sounded like it came from some big animal. I love my wife. We've been married three years. But still, the sight of her bare, but for a tiny scrap of cotton that she called underwear, called up my inner caveman.

"I heard that," she said. "Don't scare our guest."

Dan didn't so much look scared as stunned.

"I'm not scared," he managed to utter.

She walked to him and put her hand behind his head, pulling his face to her lower belly, just above her panties. "Good," she said. "Because I want you to eat me, Dan. Like you did our freshman year of college."

His eyes darted to me then, and I grinned and shrugged. "Best to give the lady what she wants."

Dan pulled her panties down, and Belinda spread her legs wider. She tilted her hips and pushed his head, and then his mouth was on her, his tongue slipping between her folds and finding her clit. Belinda ground herself against his mouth with her eyes shut and her head tossed back as she clutched two big hanks of his hair in her hands.

She thrust against his lips over and over as I heard the wet sounds of his attention. Then she climaxed, her eyes opening slowly to stare at me. I gave her a saucy wink, and she smiled.

"Unzip your pants. Sit back. Relax," she cooed, and I stood as he obeyed her instructions.

I pulled my belt free and tossed it on the chair. Then I took down my pants and my boxer briefs and moved up behind her as she dropped to her knees on the hardwood floor. She took his cock—a big cock, mind you—in her hand and began to stroke it. When he stopped looking at me and my erection and shut his eyes in surrender, she put her mouth on him. First, she sucked on only the tip of him, making him moan. Then she slid her wet, pink tongue down his cock and sucked for all she was worth.

I slipped into her pussy slowly, holding her hips and watching her little round ass under my hands. Watching my cock disappear into her never got old.

She was tight around me, and her cunt milked me so intensely that I had to focus on not coming to make the moment last. I shoved myself forward into her roughly the way she liked. The way that got her off. She groaned softly around his cock, which made him exhale loudly.

Belinda pulled back and looked at him. "Don't come. I want you in my pussy. Okay?"

He nodded fast and then she gave him a few more deep-throat sucks as I rocked my hips and fucked her smoothly. I reached beneath her and found her clit, rubbing it hard. Her button was still wet from his mouth, and the lubrication of his saliva eased the motion of my fingers. She moved in tandem with me, squeezing her cunt around me, and when I moaned, she came, shivering with delight.

Then she pulled back and sighed. "Switch, boys."

But she actually turned. Not us. She turned to wrap her lips around my hard-on and began to give me a blow job. I tugged her long red hair, using a fistful in each hand as reins. He stood behind her, and I pointed, "End table. Condoms. Use one."

Dan nodded and moved, on what appeared to be unsteady legs, to do what I'd said. When his cock was sheathed he came back, took her hips rather shyly in his hands and slid into my wife. She was so drenched from me fucking her, I knew he had to have an easy entry. The look on his face said it was.

She knew what she was doing when it came to me. Belinda loves to go down on me, and who was I to argue? She sucked hard enough to make my balls ache with a need to come, and then pulled back to rim my cockhead with her slick tongue until I thought I'd weep. She used her hands then, a fist up and down my shaft until I couldn't stand it anymore. The sight of her, the sound of her and the feel of her were overwhelming, and then add to that the sight of her ex-boyfriend banging her, and I was done.

"Open up," I instructed conversationally.

She obliged after murmuring, "Baby, baby."

When I shot my load, she managed to capture almost every drop, rubbing the remnants along her lips with her tongue before swallowing.

"Jesus…Jesus," our visitor whispered.

"Pull out," I said. He obeyed so fast I almost laughed.

I turned Belinda toward him, so he could see her small, perfect tits and her come-laced lower lip and her pretty, dazed eyes.

"Here you go. Come on her," I said. "Come on her tits and then stick that big cock in her mouth. She'll lick it clean."

She smiled, and he whimpered. My words had the desired effect. He was trembling as he pulled the condom off, and it only took three good strokes before he cussed softly and came. His cream hit her pert breasts in ropey ribbons, and he was gasping. Then she reached for him, helped him guide his dick between her Cupid's-bow lips, and she sucked him clean.

We were all breathing hard. I helped my wife stand, and then I affectionately stroked Belinda's ass and looped an arm casually around her shoulder. Dan looked stunned, and she looked amused.

"So," I said to Dan, "you want to stay for dinner?"

He looked surprised and uncertain.

"I have some ideas for dessert," Belinda said. She smiled at him, then me.

He swallowed hard, and I wasn't sure he'd go for it until he exhaled and said, "Sure, I'd love to."

We made him glad he stayed after all.

A Perfect Match

Mark Donohue

The first time I saw Larissa was outside my office building. She was standing off to the side, next to one of the outdoor ashtrays, chain-smoking her way through a pack of cigarettes. She lit her new ciga-rette off the still-burning stub of the last one, then happily inhaled, a look of pure bliss on her face. When she exhaled the smoke, her lips assumed a perfect pucker, and the smoke billowed forth in a tight stream. Every so often, she'd puff out a series of smoke rings instead, and each time her red lips parted to release them, I felt my dick throb with arousal.

I've never been much of a smoker myself, but I would light up once in a while when I wanted to check out the stunning women enjoying their cigarette breaks. It felt odd to stand in their midst without a cigarette between my lips, so I'd picked up the habit. Plus, in a crowd of smokers, it never hurt to have a pack of cigarettes and a lighter on hand just in case. You never knew when a beautiful woman would need you to relight her menthol, or when you'd be approached by someone who wanted to bum a smoke. I'd learned early on to always be prepared.

Larissa disappeared before I had a chance to approach her that first day, but over the next couple of weeks, I spotted her at least a dozen more times. Usually, we were headed in opposite directions, her on her way outside for a smoke while I was on my way back to my office. I got lucky one day and was sitting outside enjoying a cup of coffee when she came out for her morning break. She pulled a cigarette out of the pack in her hand, then fumbled around for a minute looking for her lighter, which she seemed to have misplaced. Finally, I saw my opening. I hurried to her rescue, since I always have my lighter in my pocket. She happily accepted my offer, and after she took her first relieved pull on her cigarette, I struck up a conversation.

Larissa, it turned out, worked on the same floor as me. She'd started her job about a month earlier, which is why I'd only seen her around for the past few weeks, and her schedule was slightly different from mine. But, she admitted, that didn't stop her from taking her smoking breaks at regular intervals.

As we talked, she continued puffing at her cigarette and blowing smoke trails, and I wondered if I should tell her how sexy she looked doing it. I wasn't sure how she'd take that, though, so I kept my mouth shut on the topic and instead asked her when she planned to take her next break. "Maybe we could grab lunch between cigarettes?" I suggested. She readily agreed, and a few hours later, we met up for sandwiches and smokes, and I once again got to light her cigarette and watch her blow smoke rings.

For the rest of the week, I joined Larissa on the majority of her "intermissions," as she called them, lighting her cigarettes and admiring the way her lips wrapped around the filter or puckered as she exhaled the smoke from her lungs. I was in a constant state of arousal around her, but I never could find the right time to make my move. I wasn't even sure my advances would be welcome; I couldn't read Larissa's signals to save my life.

Fortunately, on Friday afternoon, Larissa made the move for me. We were on our way out of the building at the end of the day when she pulled out a cigarette and asked me for one last light. After her cigarette was lit, she shocked me by walking away. I assumed that was it and I'd see her the following week, but she got only a few feet before turning around and asking me, "Are you coming or what?" I had no idea where she was going, but you'd better believe I was going with her.

I followed Larissa across the parking lot to her car, and then she drove us to a restaurant near her apartment. She led me to an outside table—where, she said, she could continue smoking—and then sat across from me and flagged down the waiter to get us menus. We had a nice dinner, sharing the delicious Italian fare and a bottle of Chardonnay, and talking about our lives and jobs. Then, over dessert, she shocked me again.

As she blew rings of smoke up into the air, she looked at me and said, "I've seen you watching me. You like when I smoke, don't you?" I nodded. "I've only seen you smoke twice," she continued, "yet you're always outside on the smokers' patio, and you always have a lighter or pack of cigarettes on hand. Has anyone else ever caught on to your dirty little fetish?" I told her they hadn't, and she smiled. Then she invited me back to her place. "I have a comfy bed and a whole carton of smokes," she told me, then pointed across the street as she said, "And I live right over there."

I paid the bill and then followed Larissa across the street, up the stairs and into her fourth-floor apartment. She kissed me once we crossed over the threshold, and she tasted bitter and smoky, a delicious flavor combination. Her lips were firm but pliant, and her tongue eagerly fought mine in an arousing battle for control of our kiss. My cock was pants-splittingly hard after watching her smoke all day, and when she rubbed up against me, I nearly came from the contact. I couldn't remember the last time I'd been so turned on.

Our game of tongue-tag continued as we ground our pelvises together and felt each other up. However, we both became desperate for release. We didn't even make it to the bedroom, instead stripping each other right there in the living room and collapsing naked onto her plush leather sofa. Larissa was on top, and she seemed to relish being in the driver's seat. She straddled my hips, her soft thighs wrapping around my body, then grabbed my dick and guided my hard-on into her hot, wet center. As she sank down on me, she started to rock back and forth, fucking herself with my stiff cock. It felt so good, after a week of foreplay, to finally be inside her pussy, and I knew I would reach my climax in record time.

While Larissa continued to ride me, I started to thrust into her, matching her stroke for stroke. Soon we had a steady rhythm going, and I felt her pussy begin to pulse around my shaft. I knew she was getting close, and I wasn't far behind, either. It wouldn't be long before our orgasms hit.

A few minutes later, I felt Larissa's pussy clench and release my dick repeatedly, and then I felt a gush of warm fluid as she came around my shaft. A split second after that, I came, firing my load up into her. We continued to move together as we climaxed, and we didn't stop until we were both completely spent. Then Larissa collapsed on top of me and I felt her chest moving against mine as we breathed heavily in the aftermath of our intense climaxes.

As soon as Larissa's breathing evened out, she wriggled around so that she was leaning over the edge of the sofa. Then she reached across to the coffee table, where I noticed a half-empty pack of cigarettes, a book of matches and an ashtray. She shook a cigarette out of the pack as she handed me the matches, and I lit the end for her as she sucked in through the filter. In a flash, there was a tantalizing trail of smoke slipping out between her soft pink lips, and this time, I knew she was doing it just for me.

Pretty Little Hand-Me-Downs

ANGELO VITALE

My wife has a rule that whenever she buys something new, she has to get rid of something old to make room for it. I appreciate this rule most when my wife goes shopping for new clothes, because it means that I get her cast-offs for myself. Although I'm a few inches taller and have broader shoulders, Kristin has a strong, athletic build, so her clothes often fit me, if a little more snug than appropriate.

When she came home on Saturday afternoon, laden with shopping bags, I got excited. Kristin breezed past me and went straight for the bedroom, barely greeting me, but I didn't care. All I cared about was finding out what pretty little hand-me-downs I'd be getting once she was done unpacking all her overflowing bags. I thought I'd have to wait awhile before Kristin let me see her haul—and mine—but after only a few short minutes, she called me into the bedroom.

She was standing in front of the closet, a half-dozen dresses hanging over her left arm as she flipped through the rack of clothing in front of her; a pile of silk and lace lingerie sat on the bed behind her. I knew that soon those discarded clothes would be mine, and I ogled them longingly.

"I have something special for you," Kristin said. She added the load of dresses she was holding to the growing pile of clothing on the bed and came over to me. She leaned over to kiss me, then reached behind me to grab one of the large shopping bags. She peeked inside, then pulled it around and handed it to me. "I got this for you," she told me. "It's been a while since you've had something all your own, and I thought you deserved something new."

I reached in and pulled out several items, each wrapped in a thin sheet of white tissue paper. Only the nicest stores did that sort of thing, so I knew right away that my gift was going to be exceptional. I carefully peeled up the tape on the first package and unfolded the paper, revealing a pair of lace bikini panties and a matching bra. The next package contained a pair of silk stockings with thick black seams running up the backs. Then there was a garter belt. Finally, I unwrapped the last item, a dark blue pencil dress with small cap sleeves and some ruching on the right side by the waist; it was absolutely beautiful. Even better, though, is that the dress was in my size, not Kristin's. I stared at it, dumbstruck. Kristin usually buys me something for my birthday or holidays, but never a full ensemble at once, and never anything so extravagant. My cock pulsed in my pants as I fingered the garment. I couldn't believe my luck.

Smiling, Kristin told me, "Help me put away the rest of your things and then we can hop in the shower. You know, those new clothes will feel so much better on a squeaky-clean body."

I didn't have to be told twice. I gathered up all the clothes she'd discarded and raced to put them away in the closet in my office, where I keep all my feminine attire. By the time everything was in its place, steam was pouring out of the master bathroom, and I got there just in time to see Kristin disappear into the shower.

I quickly shed my clothing, tossed it into the hamper and stepped into the shower with my wife. She was already standing under the spray, and I watched as the hot water streamed over her toned, curvy body. I traced the water's path with my eyes, following the rivulets as they raced down her neck and shoulders and over her small, firm breasts. She had her head tipped back and eyes closed as she wet her hair, but when she opened them again, her gaze traveled over me straight to my throbbing erection. She was on her knees a second later, the head of my shaft between her lips.

Her tongue swirled around the tip of my cock before she sucked me deeper into her mouth, and I felt my shaft throb. I bucked my hips forward, wanting her to take me farther into her throat, and she opened wide. I continued thrusting back and forth, fucking her mouth, and when I felt my balls tighten, I squeezed her shoulder to let her know that I was about to come. She didn't stop sucking, and a minute later, as her tongue pressed against the underside of my shaft, I shot my load into her mouth.

After I'd climaxed, Kristin released my cock and stood up, and we continued our shower. Kristin poured some of her lavender shampoo into her hands and massaged some into my hair, then started washing her own. Then she rubbed her bar of moisturizing soap onto her loofah and started scrubbing me with it. She worked from my shoulders all the way down to my toes, moving the sponge in soft circles all over my body. When she was done, I took the loofah from her and returned the gesture, generously soaping her curves. I even snuck a hand between her thighs and briefly fingered her warm, wet pussy.

Once we were done, we toweled off and took turns using the blow-dryer. Then, standing side by side in front of the large bathroom mirror, we carefully applied our makeup. Our movements were almost synchronized as we first put on tinted moisturizer and then used the wands from our concealer to cover up some small skin imperfections. Kristin then applied a cream blush, while I used a little bronzer, the way she'd taught me, to create the appearance of cheekbones. After that came eye shadow, liner and mascara, and finally some bright-red lipstick for us both.

At last, it was time to get dressed, and we returned to the bedroom to slip into our new outfits. While Kristin dug through her bags to find just the right thing to wear, I began to put on the lingerie she'd bought me. I pulled on the small pink panties first, wiggling a bit to get them over my hardening cock, then strapped the dainty bra across my chest. The stockings were next, and I scrunched the first one down to the toes before carefully pulling it up my leg, being sure to keep the seam straight as I attached it to the garter belt. Then I repeated the process with the other stocking, until both legs were encased in smooth silk up to the thigh.

I turned to admire myself in the mirror on the door of my wife's closet, and when I did, I saw Kristin already in her short red cocktail dress. She looked sexy as hell. I gave her a once-over, admiring the way the dress's square neckline showcased her cleavage while the length of the skirt was perfect for displaying her long, lean legs. Kristin looked me up and down, too, her eyes lingering on the bulge in the front of my lacy panties. I knew I looked good, but while she ogled me, I turned my head to check myself out in the mirror again. I got so distracted by my reflection that I didn't notice Kristin inching forward until she was right on top of me, her hand rubbing my dick through the lace.

She palmed my hardening shaft and then lightly caressed it with her fingertips, moving them slowly up and down my length. My dick was rock hard again in a matter of moments. She stroked me a few more times, then pushed the panty crotch to the side until my cock was free and jutting out from my body. The lace scratched against my shaft, producing an incredible sensation. It felt so good, but I knew that there was something else that would feel even better.

I pulled Kristin closer and reached under her dress to pull down her panties, but I discovered that she wasn't wearing any. I rubbed my hand along her slit for a few seconds, and then led her toward the bed. I pushed her onto her back, pulled the bottom of her dress up to expose her cunt, and then climbed on top of her. I jerked my cock a few times in my fist, making sure I was ready to go, then guided my dick into her waiting pussy. She was slick and hot, and as I slid inside her, my dick throbbed with my desire. I waited a minute, savoring her heat, then started thrusting. As I moved, the layers of tulle under her dress rubbed against my bare skin, and the sensation drove me crazy, making me pump faster.

I loved the feeling of my lace panties scratching along my cock and the tulle from her dress rubbing against my stomach. The silk of my stockings caressed my legs as I fucked Kristin, and the satin bodice of her dress felt smooth as my chest pressed against hers. All of our feminine finery felt so delicious against my skin, so arousing.

I always come incredibly fast when I'm dressed in drag, and that night was no different. Kristin shifted on the bed, bringing her knees up and planting her feet flat on the mattress, allowing me to go even deeper insider her. I pushed myself up on my arms, giving me more leverage, then started to really pound her, thrusting as hard and as fast and as deep as I could.

A few more thrusts, and I was done. I felt my balls tighten and my cock throb, and then I exploded, shooting my load deep into my wife's clenching cunt. While I poured my seed into her, Kristin reached between our bodies and started playing with her clit, frantically frigging the hard button until she came, too.

Both sated, we sat up, shared a sweet kiss, and then finished getting ready for our dress-up date. Kristin touched up her makeup and styled her hair while I slipped into my brand-new dress. It was still early, so we had plenty of time for dinner and drinks—and another bedroom romp, too.

Doing Things Differently

SARAH JACKSON

We all decided to swap. There were four of us, and over dinner one night, John and Bob started joking about it. Then more wine was poured, and we all started to discuss it in earnest. Us swapping. Mary going with my husband, John, and me going with Bob. We set a date before the night was over, and then John took me upstairs and fucked me until my knees were weak.

I really thought we'd call it off. I never thought we'd go through with it. Not until the night came and they arrived. Me and Bob to go off to one hotel, John and Mary to go off to another. We wanted neutral locations to act out our fantasies.

John kissed me goodbye, tweaked my nipple through my wrap dress, and whispered, "Have fun, be safe. I love you."

At the hotel, I was a bundle of nerves. I wandered the lavish lobby while Bob checked us in. Then he was at my side, gripping my elbow lightly and whispering in my ear, "Time to go up. Are you ready?"

I swallowed hard but managed to nod. I didn't think my voice would comply if I tried to speak.

We were alone on the elevator, and Bob, much bigger and broader than my John, pushed me to the back right corner and brought his lips to my own. His kiss was demanding, his tongue stroking boldly over mine. He gripped my hips and slid my dress up some so it sat high on my thighs. He'd positioned us so the obvious security camera was pointed right at us—at me pushed in a corner being manhandled and groped by someone other than my husband.

Wetness streaked my panties, and lust roared through my belly and my cunt. I was breathless.

When the doors popped open and he led me out into the hallway, I was mindless with lust.

Inside the hotel room, I stood in the center of the lush space and waited. Bob circled me like a shark. My nipples felt tight and sensitive against the bodice of my dress. He stopped directly behind me, put his mouth to the back of my neck, and my skin prickled with energy and arousal.

"What does he do to you?" he asked.

I blinked, my brain trying to unscramble what sounded to my ears like a riddle. "What?"

"What does he do to you? John. Tell me."

As he spoke, his hands skimmed my sides, his touch igniting the skin beneath the thin black-and-taupe fabric of my dress. He cupped my breasts. He didn't pinch or stroke my nipples; no, he simply held me in his hands and waited for me to speak, with his warm lips still pressed to my nape.

"I...he goes down on me. Almost always." I laughed shrilly, feeling so stupid but also, oh so turned on. "To get me ready," I resumed, my voice warbling. "And then he pushes me back and kisses me until I'm desperate and then he enters me."

Heat rushed to my cheeks as I finished that sentence.

"Face-to-face?" His tongue slid along the tender spot where my neck met my shoulder, and I shivered.

"What?"

"Does your husband fuck you face-to-face?"

"Al...almost always," I stammered as Bob's big hands began to tug at the bow that held my wrap dress shut.

"Good to know. Thank you, sweetheart." Then he pulled hard enough that the belt came undone and the dress sagged open.

Bob peeled the dress off me, then unhooked my bra and removed that, too. I stood there, docile and panting for breath, as he undressed me. He walked me to the mirror by pushing his chest and cock to my back and ass. When we faced the large, ornate mirror, he pulled my panties down and tossed them aside. Looking over my shoulder, his dark eyes pinned me in a mesmerizing gaze.

"Watch me," he said. "I want to do things different than you're used to."

He wrapped his arms around my waist as I watched and then pulled my nether lips back to expose me. I stared, barely breathing, as he began to stroke my clit rhythmically. Every few seconds, he'd bite my earlobe, the side of my neck, the slope of my shoulder, keeping me off balance and dizzy with want.

His fingers slipped back farther, teasing my opening and gathering moisture. His left hand slipped up to cup my breast, his fingers pinching my nipple hard enough to make me gasp.

He drove his fingers into me, but only briefly, and then stroked my clit harder than I'd ever think to. I came, trembling in his arms. His dark eyes seemed darker in our reflection. His smile was wicked.

He pushed me so that I had to put my hands against the dresser below the mirror. I watched him in the glass as he found a condom and rolled it on. My pussy beat in time with my pulse, and I wondered if my knees would hold me. I'd stopped wondering if I'd go through with it and began to wonder if I could handle it.

"Spread your legs," he said softly.

I spread them wider than they were and waited, my skin cool with anticipation as he moved in behind me. Making sure to watch me the whole time, Bob ran his cock from my ass to my slit to my clit and then back again, keeping me on edge, keeping me waiting.

I hung my head, desperate to focus on anything but my wild desire. However, he tapped my bottom with his hand, not hard enough to be a slap but definitely hard enough to get my attention.

"Eyes up. Attention on us."

I immediately looked back up. I wondered wildly if John was fucking Mary face-to-face, missionary-style. A small laugh burst out of me; I couldn't contain it.

"Care to share?" Before I could answer, he slipped the head of his cock into me. His fingers dug into my hips, and I heard myself sigh deeply. Then he thrust into me fast and hard, and I moaned. "Never mind," he said softly, pinching my nipple again. "Forget I asked."

My body rocked as he fucked me. I was pliant and soft, his

willing puppet as he kept me bent at the angle he liked best. Every stroke of his cock deep inside was echoed by an almost-too-gentle stroke of his finger over my clit. At random times he'd pinch my nipple and I'd jump in his arms.

"You seem to like this." He bit my shoulder roughly, and I found myself coming again, shaking hard in his embrace.

Bob stopped talking. He simply growled and pushed his hand to the small of my back. I leaned forward more, bending to his will, and ground back against him as he thrust deeply into me. His movements became rougher, more desperate, and I found myself squeezing my internal muscles around him.

"Fuck," he hissed, and then he was coming, his face serious and handsome. I watched him, mesmerized as he finished.

He smiled at me in the mirror. "Are you okay?"

I could only nod.

"Up for the rest of our night together?"

I felt dizzy at the prospect of the night ahead. "Yes."

"Good. I have a lot of things I want us to try together. And I don't want to waste a single minute."

We didn't waste a single minute, and a few times a year we still head off to separate hotels. Me with Bob, John with Mary. It works well for us. We look forward to it.

Taken for a Ride

VANCE PETERMAN

When Terry told me she was going to ride in the limo to Bob and Judy's wedding because she was one of the bridesmaids, I felt hopeful. We'd long had a fantasy that we'd been dying to try out, and seeing how the limo driver had been admiring my wife, it looked like this could be our chance.

The ceremony was a long, stuffy affair and the entire time I watched the wedding party up at the altar, all I could think about was the driver—a big, strapping guy with a shorn head and tattoos that were visible beneath the cuffs of his white shirt. I shut my eyes while the vows were being said, picturing him with my slim, gorgeous Terry. She'd managed to make the sea-foam-green bridesmaid dress look good, and that was saying something.

I had to put the thought of watching them out of my mind, or I'd end up with a full-blown hard-on in the middle of church.

Afterward, it seemed to take forever to get to the reception, but I finally arrived and managed to find a parking spot. Inside, the music was already pounding, the liquor was flowing and I spotted Terry doing a crazy dance with the other bridesmaids. She waved and hurried over to talk to me. She tugged me into the coatroom and whispered in my ear, "Did you see him?"

I nodded, unable to speak because I was already so turned on.

"He's perfect, isn't he?"

Instead of answering, I glanced around to make sure we were alone before taking her hand and placing her palm on my erection. I wished she were actually touching me—and not through my dress pants—but just the pressure of her hand there was wonderful.

"I know. Give me half an hour, and then follow me out—okay? I'll leave once the toasts are done."

I nodded, and she kissed me, slipping her tongue into my mouth briefly before hurrying back to the party. I never thought I'd survive the toasts, but finally they ended and I saw her give me a tiny wave and then rush outside.

I gave her only ten minutes, and then made my way to the parking lot. I crept up by the side of the limo and peeked inside. My heart lurched, and my cock grew even more rigid when I saw her through the cracked window. The windows of the vehicle were tinted, so she told me she'd have him open one slightly so I could see inside. She'd done as promised. That's my girl.

Terry was down on her knees between his spread thighs. The driver had his hand settled possessively on her blonde hair as she sucked him off. Her dress was still on, but it was a puddle of sea foam around her lower body. She sucked him eagerly, her head bobbing up and down as small grunts and sighs came from her.

I wanted to touch my cock but was afraid to. The visual was just too good—after so many hours fantasizing and talking about her screwing another man, she was taking the plunge. And if I touched myself, I thought I might come instantly and give myself away with my orgasmic groans. I was afraid to breathe, let alone jerk off.

She pulled her mouth off his dick with an audible pop and began to stroke his length with her fist. Terry kissed her way down his balls, sucking each one enthusiastically as he groaned, raising his hips to get better contact with her talented mouth.

"Take off that dress, sweetheart."

"But what if my husband comes?" Terry asked, and I almost smiled. She was teasing me.

"It's not him coming I'm worried about," the driver said.

She crouched in the back of the limo and took off her dress after he helped with her zipper.

The music from the reception boomed; the bass seemed to rumble up through my feet into my groin. I bit my lower lip to sharpen my focus.

She pushed her ass back to the driver, and he helped her peel off her panties. I held my breath as he delved into her from behind, licking her pussy with noisy groans. She leaned back, her face toward me as she pinched and stroked her nipples. For all I knew, she could see me watching at the opening she'd provided.

"That's it, baby," he said, easing back and appearing as if he was worming his finger into her asshole. Then he tugged her toward him.

"Got a condom?" Terry queried. That was her rule. No protection, no fucking.

He practically broke his own arm getting his wallet out of his pants. She rolled the rubber on for him, her body wedged between his thighs again. Her bare ass was pointed my way, and I could see wetness where his mouth had been.

When he was sheathed, she knelt on the seat between his knees, pressing her tits to his mouth. He took a nipple between his teeth and tugged so that the puckered skin stretched out and she moaned. Then he repeated the same action on the other breast. Terry moaned again.

He grunted, "Get up here. Get on my cock."

Terry stood and turned toward me, then lowered her body. She slid herself down on his hard length and shivered as she settled in. His arm wrapped around her belly, his mouth found her shoulder, and then when she began to move rhythmically, he thrust upward.

His hands found her beautiful breasts, and he played with her erect nipples until her motions grew more ragged and urgent. I watched her thrust her hips and grind, watched as her breath grew short. She came with her hands pressed to the limo ceiling and the driver praising her tight little cunt.

He didn't come, though, and she licked her lips, her gaze sliding to the barely open window as she lowered herself back between his legs, ripped off the condom and sucked him until he was yanking twin portions of her honey-colored hair with his big hands.

When he cried out, thrusting his hips up hard, she pulled back and jerked his cock furiously. His come shot across her breasts and her shoulders. With her free hand, she smeared his cream down her belly as he watched. One more jerk emptied him fully. His eyes went heavy with pleasure, and he laughed softly.

"Well, you were a real nice surprise."

She smiled. "Thanks. I had fun. But now I have to go. I have someone in there saving a dance for me."

I took my cue to leave, hurrying back across the parking lot to get inside. I was thankful my jacket was long enough to cover my erection. I had a feeling it wouldn't be going anywhere for a while.

When she reappeared with roses in her cheeks and her hair wild, I was waiting with a drink.

"Did you enjoy that?" she whispered against my ear. I wrapped my arms around her and began to sway to the slow song. She pressed against me, felt my hard-on and smiled. "Or do I even have to ask?"

"I loved it," I said, embracing her even closer. When she moved against me, I wondered if for the first time in a decade I was at risk of coming in my pants.

"Good, because when this song is over, there's something I'd like to show you in the coatroom."

"What's that?" I asked.

"How fast I can make that dick of yours go from hard to soft by making you come."

I pictured that pretty painted mouth of hers on my cock right after it had been on another man's and had to suppress a groan of pleasure. "It's a date," I said, and kissed her.